BUILDING A LIGHT

MY PHYSICAL THERAPY RESIDENCY JOURNEY THROUGH COVID-19

DEREK TAO

Copyright © 2024 by Derek Tao
All rights reserved.

No part of this publication may be reproduced, distributed, or transmitted in any form or by any means, including photocopying, recording, or other electronic or mechanical methods, without the prior written permission of the author, except as permitted by U.S. copyright law and for use of quotations in a book review. For permission requests, contact Derek Tao at dtao800@gmail.com

Book and Cover Design by Stewart Williams
Edited by Jennifer Watson

First Edition, 2024
Published by Derek Tao

Available in print formats through Ingram Spark,
Amazon and Barnes & Noble Press
ISBN: 979-8-9915349-0-1 (Ingram Spark)
ISBN: 979-8-9915349-1-8 (Amazon)
ISBN: 979-8-9915349-2-5 (Barnes & Noble Press)

Available in digital formats through Amazon,
Apple Books and Barnes & Noble
ISBN: 979-8-9915349-3-2 (Amazon Kindle)
ISBN: 979-8-9915349-4-9 (Apple Books)
ISBN: 979-8-9915349-5-6 (Barnes & Noble)

For more information or inquiries, email dtao800@gmail.com

Dedicated to physical therapy residents and their patients, each navigating life's uncertainties on a mutual journey with different perspectives.

*To protect the privacy of the patients and professionals described herein, some of the names have been changed.

"A candle burns away with each passing moment. Yet, within these moments, it dispels the darkness with its light."

The Light in Each Moment, p. 2

TABLE OF CONTENTS

INTRODUCTION IX

PROLOGUE. XIV

THE FIRST TRIMESTER 1

   Welcome to Residency. 3
   Mentoring Introductions 7
   The World of Telehealth. 13
   Introducing Students to Clinical Practice 23
   The Ripple Effect of Politics. 27
   The First Live Patient Examination (LPE) 32
   A Dark Winter Ahead. 42

THE SECOND TRIMESTER. 45

   New Year, New Learning Curve 47
   Hope 53
   Never a Dull Moment 57
   Atlanta 68
   The Second LPE 71

THE THIRD TRIMESTER 77

   The Second Live Patient Examination, Round 2. 79
   The Second Technique Practical Exam and Written Exam. . . . 86
   Digging Through Fog 90
   Remembering Why I Started 95
   The Final Live Patient Examination 101
   Goodbyes and Graduation 110
   The Last Day 116

EPILOGUE 118

ACKNOWLEDGMENTS. 124

BIBLIOGRAPHY 127

ENDNOTES. 130

INTRODUCTION

"The purpose of going on a long journey is to learn more about yourself."

When I was in high school, I took an Honors English class with a memorable teacher. I only remember bits and pieces about the books we read, but one of the most memorable things he told our class, was the quote above. In the books we analyzed, the main characters would often embark on various journeys, and whether intended or not, they would learn something about themselves. Sometimes it was positive, other times not so much. The characters were seldom the exact same version of themselves by the end of the book.

People throughout time have embarked on journeys for various reasons, and by the end of those journeys, it changed them: deeply and meaningfully.

When an individual makes a conscious choice to embark on a journey; pushing the absolute limits of themselves in one dimension of life or other, they then have the opportunity to enter a unique stratosphere where they can learn some very interesting and pivotal lessons about themselves, about the people around them, about the world they live in, and about the world at large. This can be applied to many facets of life, including but not limited to athletics, academics, careers, and more. For my journey, we are interested in the realm of healthcare, and more specifically, of physical therapy.

This is the story of an emerging healthcare provider making the conscious choice to embark on a year-long journey of professional

INTRODUCTION

growth amidst the uncertainty of a global pandemic. This is the story of an orthopedic physical therapy resident.

∿

What is a physical therapy residency? Well, to define this on a surface level, we must first ask: What is physical therapy? What is a residency?

If you search online through Merriam-Webster's Dictionary, one can find the following definitions:

Physical therapy

(referred to as physiotherapy outside of the US)

- therapy that is used to preserve, enhance, or restore movement and physical function impaired or threatened by disease, injury, or disability and that utilizes therapeutic exercise, physical modalities (such as massage and electrotherapy), assistive devices, and patient education and training.[1]

Physical Therapist

(referred to as physiotherapist outside of the US)

- a health care professional who provides therapy to preserve, enhance, or restore movement and physical function that are impaired or threatened by disease, injury, or disability.[2]

Residency

- a period of advanced training in a medical specialty that normally follows graduation from medical school and licensing to practice medicine.[3]

When people go through physical therapy, their initial visit usually starts off with an evaluation where the patient and physical therapist discuss a patient's reasons for seeking out physical therapy, the physical therapist performs a physical examination of the patient, and then the physical therapist provides recommendations for treatment based on the examination findings. Subsequent visits with a physical therapist involve updating the physical therapist on changes to their condition and continuation of care. The patient is followed throughout their care, and as additional information is gathered through successive consultations, the physical therapist will continuously update treatment to match the needs of the patient accordingly.

The American Physical Therapy Association, or APTA, reports that as of 2019, there are 312,716 licensed physical therapists in the United States.[4] The American Board of Physical Therapy Specialties reports on their website that as of June 2023, 37,752 physical therapists are Board certified as clinical specialists.[5] While both numbers have grown since, it is most likely estimated that only approximately 10% of all physical therapists are Board certified specialists. Of the specialties, the most common one is Orthopedics, which focuses on neuromusculoskeletal care.

To become a physical therapist in the US at present, one must have a bachelor's degree, and then undergo a three-year graduate school program.[6] Upon graduation, physical therapists are granted a doctorate degree and permission to take the necessary licensure exams. Students must pass the National Physical Therapy Examination, or NPTE. In certain States of the US, a jurisprudence exam is also required which assesses one's knowledge of the laws and regulations related to the practice of physical therapy in said State. Once licensed, physical therapists may enter the workforce directly to treat patients.

Medical residencies are commonly associated with the postgraduate specialty training that physicians undergo after graduating from medical school to develop the necessary foundational clinical

INTRODUCTION

expertise needed to treat patients. Residencies for other medical professions have become increasingly common with the goal of enhancing the quality of care provided. This was the inspiration for physical therapy residencies around the US to be established and developed. While physical therapists are not required to complete a residency in order to practice, a residency provides a structured opportunity for mentorship, rapid professional growth and personal introspection that may not occur otherwise. Residencies for physicians range from 3 years to 7 years. In contrast, physical therapy residencies are 1 year.

I believe that the surface level technical definitions listed above only capture a partial dimension of what it means to be a physical therapist and what it means to be a resident. The healthcare field is a unique environment where humanity intersects. It is a profession where one has the opportunity to meet people from all different backgrounds and places. It is a place where I can work with someone who is a retired award-winning author, and on the same day work with someone struggling to make ends meet with rent. It is a convergence where people come for help, a space where people find solace, a connection where people find hope. It is a place where people laugh, cry, celebrate, cringe, worry and learn. The unique position of healthcare presents the chance for providers to bring a metaphorical *light* to the lives of patients, serving as a figurative *beacon,* illuminating a path for navigating seemingly uncertain health challenges. With the nature of physical therapy, it is common for people to attend multiple sessions over time, allowing for a meaningful relationship to grow between a physical therapist and a patient; between two people working together on a journey. Like a bridge being built to span a river: patient and provider build something altogether new with their slow but methodical combined efforts.

As I embarked on my journey as a new physical therapy res-

INTRODUCTION

ident, navigating my first year of clinical practice, I sought *not only* to try to bring a metaphorical *light* to each clinical encounter. Simultaneously, I sought to build the capacity of that *light* through my personal growth as a clinician and person. Along the way, I kept a journal where I wrote about the journey, and it has served as both inspiration for this book and a continuing exploration of the struggles and triumphs of a physical therapy resident navigating his first year of clinical practice in an uncertain world.

PROLOGUE

I suppose a bit of background for how I ended up on this particular life trajectory would be useful here. Growing up, I did not know physical therapy existed until my last year of high school. I was not even interested in anything healthcare related until that year. I am a competitive runner and back then, had been running cross country and track for many years for school teams. Throughout my early running career, I struggled a lot with different injuries. My mother would always tell me to rest from those injuries, and most of the time, rest was sufficient to heal the injuries. However, when I sustained a hip injury in my last year of high school that led to swelling inside my hip joint, despite resting for almost six weeks, it did not improve. Frustration sank in as I struggled to cope with this loss of freedom, and some nights, I cried myself to sleep to escape my feelings of hopelessness. I visited multiple physicians and specialists, but none of them were able to give me a conclusive answer that would help me to properly treat my injury and return to running. My coach and one of my teammates both recommended that I go to physical therapy, and since my injury was not improving, my mother agreed to bring me.

Going to see a physical therapist was a profound, eye-opening experience. The therapist I saw empathized with me, as he had also sustained injuries before through playing sports and understood how difficult it was to not be able to do something I genuinely enjoyed. He also assured me that my condition would improve, and I felt very supported in my rehabilitation goals of working

PROLOGUE

back towards returning to competitive running. Gradually, over the course of 4 months, my condition improved. During this time, whenever I went in to get treatment, I would note how my physical therapist would empathize with other patients and how patients responded to that empathy with optimism about their rehabilitation. I swapped stories with other patients, and they had all kinds of injuries. There was one thing that everyone had in common though: the hopeful feeling of reassurance felt by everyone through the physical therapist's empathy, skill, and thoughtful care. Through my experiences and through speaking with other patients, I saw with physical therapy something that I had not seen before in my experiences with other healthcare providers up to this point in life: the opportunity to closely connect with patients while empowering them to return to living their lives.

This experience of being a patient in physical therapy was a time when a healthcare provider shared a figurative light for me, a place to hold hope in a fairytale athletics comeback and to dream of returning to doing something again that I loved to do. I am a firm believer that the things that have happened to me in my life occur with intentional reason for a greater purpose, and although it quite sucked having that hip injury, I eventually successfully got healthy and discovered a career path that gave me the chance to potentially pass on the figurative *light* to others.

Through my undergraduate studies and graduate level physical therapy education, I continued to have more experiences that affirmed my decision to pursue physical therapy as a career choice. I did not know that physical therapy residencies existed however until the beginning of my second year of physical therapy school. I was catching up with some of my good friends in my cohort as we were all fresh off our first clinical rotations for school. Two of my friends had completed their rotations at places that had established orthopedic physical therapy residencies, and it was eye-opening to hear them talk about their experiences with getting a taste of residency level clinical training. It became something that I considered as a post-school option, although I was not sure yet if I would commit.

As I continued to progress through physical therapy school and work my way through my third and final year of my program, I concluded that I wanted to enter the realm of orthopedics for my clinical practice. I still held reservations regarding entering a residency, however. On one hand, residency would only be one year, and it would help to significantly accelerate my growth as a clinician. On the other hand, I knew that residency would be incredibly exhausting, and I was already feeling both apprehensive and burnt out from the cumulative demands of school. I decided to keep my options relatively open and go through the application process. By the time I reached February of 2020, I had narrowed my possible post-school paths to three options. One option was applying for orthopedic residency. A second option was applying to work with a start-up company, and a third option was just to go and work at an outpatient physical therapy clinic. Each option had its pros and cons.

With the decision-making process, I reflected a lot on the theme of choosing to become either a "big fish in a small pond," vs. a "little fish in a big pond." I had to really reflect on whether I wanted to just have a small vision now or a bigger vision down the road. When taking the time to reflect on residency, I had to acknowledge that this was the most challenging option of the three, but also the one that would lead to the most growth, the one that would lead towards the bigger vision. I also hoped from the outset, that my career trajectory would move beyond patient care, to include teaching and mentoring future generations of clinicians. While residency seemed daunting, I ultimately concluded that I would have to gather the courage to rise to this challenge and to do so with the heart of dedicating myself for the betterment of others. With my reflections on my options having put residency into perspective, I felt empowered to fully commit. I submitted my application at the beginning of March, 2020, interviewed for the residency mid-April, 2020, and received an official offer at the beginning of May, 2020.

As I went through the residency application submission process and began my final clinical rotation for school, the COVID-19 pandemic unfolded globally. At first, I did not think much of it, as cases and deaths were relatively low in the United States. Within a matter of weeks, however, clinical care at my rotation site came almost to a standstill as the healthcare field came to grasp the dark storm descending upon the country and the world. News from New York began to pour in of people dying by the thousands.[7] Stories from hospitals that were becoming severely overwhelmed with patients flooded the news feeds, accompanied by haunting photos of exhausted healthcare workers donned in trash bags as makeshift protective gear and week-old masks while trying to triage patients.[8,9] It was clear that the healthcare field that I worked in was going to change very rapidly. Many students across the country were having their final rotations halted, with no definite timeline as to when they could finish. In-person care became almost non-existent at my rotation site as the regional hospital system scrambled to transition towards virtual telehealth care.

As telehealth care volume began to pick up, I had the opportunity to continue my clinical rotation and treat patients. An elevated air of anxiety seemed to be present with many clinical encounters as patients would discuss the state of the country with my clinical instructors and myself. It was certainly a very different world from what I thought I would be entering a few years ago. I was fortunate in that I was able to finish my rotation on time, but the pandemic was far from over. As the late summer approached, I knew that I would be entering residency during an ongoing pandemic. While I certainly wasn't going to be as close to treating patients with

PROLOGUE

COVID-19 as those in the ER and the ICU, I was still going to be at much higher risk of exposure to COVID-19 than someone with the option to work fully remote from home. The end of Summer 2020 had arrived, marked with licensure exams, onboarding logistics, and final moments of rest before preparing to embark on the first stage of my career as a physical therapy resident.

PART 1

The First Trimester

CHAPTER 1

Welcome to Residency

September 2020

The first week was orientation week. I thought it would only be observation of care and logistical discussions regarding expectations for the residency and such. Because of the nature of the ongoing pandemic, to enter the clinic, there was a screening checkpoint at the building ground level. Everyone that entered was required to wear a mask, all staff had to answer a pre-screening questionnaire, and all visitors were screened at the front. This was to be the daily routine for the rest of the entire residency year, a constant reminder of the pervasiveness of the COVID-19 virus.

Undergoing residency with me was none other than my trusty physical therapy school classmate, Mariano. Born in Chile and raised in the Bay Area of Northern California, Mariano brought to the dynamic a laid-back life approach paired with the ability to work hard and flow with adversity. An adventurous one at heart, he embarked on a multi-year bike trip through Brazil with his martial arts instructor prior to PT school. He was certainly the more adventurous of the two of us, and the overall contribution added some good quality to our working dynamic.

Mariano and I met with the residency coordinator Cathy, the residency director Alison, and familiarized ourselves with other residency faculty members and clinicians. The introductions were relatively smooth as there were clinicians on-site we had met as graduate students. On our lunch break, as Mariano and I waited for the elevator to go down to the ground level, he turned to me. "Dude! We're Residents!" The excitement of the year long journey ahead was evident and caused me to reflect back on my life trajectory: I had dreamed of working as a physical therapist for 8 years and was now finally starting my career! Admittedly, the start of my career had panned out quite differently from what I had imagined 8 years ago or even 3 years ago, but often life unfolds in ways that we do not expect. Mariano and I both knew the year ahead would be filled with many challenges, but his ability to take a step back and express excitement in the midst of so much uncertainty is something I'll always remember.

As part of the introductions, Cathy informed Mariano and I that we would each follow around a clinician later in the week to get a sense of clinic flow. We were informed that this would only be observation. On Friday of the first week, I was scheduled to observe one of the senior clinicians, Chris, for an evaluation. We were already acquainted, as he had helped teach a course in our PT program on the topic of specialized populations mixed with hands-on manual therapy techniques. For one day of class, I had volunteered to perform a hands-on treatment technique known as a high velocity low amplitude mobilization, and Chris volunteered to be my patient. At the time, the idea of having our professor be the subject was nerve-wracking. There was certainly no place to hide or fake the technique that I was going to do. After two failed attempts at the technique and feeling rather stressed, I decided to commit to a third attempt and in my final attempt, I succeeded on that attempt.

Back in the present, Chris and I sat in front of a desktop computer, reviewing the medical charts for the patients that I was going to observe. As we sat at the computer, Chris said to me,

"You know, I will never forget the time you cracked my back in front of your entire class and how you owned it. That's what this residency is going to be *allll* about: getting as uncomfortable as possible and *owning it!* That's what's going to make you grow." It was a great early reminder of the power of stepping outside my comfort zone. In fact, Chris already felt he knew me because at one point he watched me take that unsteady step as a student, and he remembered me for persisting despite multiple failed attempts and succeeding at the very end.

True to those words, I was going to be getting out of my comfort zone really quickly. Our next patient to be evaluated arrived for their post-surgery evaluation. They had very high energy and spunk, more than I was expecting for an early Friday morning. They also had zero filter as I would learn very quickly. This patient was already familiar with Chris, so Chris introduced me:

"This is Derek, our new ortho resident. He's going to do your exam."

Surprise!

Here I was on orientation week being thrown straight off the deep end into patient care. I didn't have a chance to refresh fully yet on my clinical examination skills and was very, very rusty. Welcome to Residency.

I proceeded through my first evaluation. It unfolded as a mess as I tried to ask questions and the patient jumped in multiple times to cut me off and give me feedback. In the process, I found out that my patient was a residency trained physical therapist who was extremely keen on giving me feedback throughout the entire encounter.

BUILDING A LIGHT

If there was an episode of Undercover Boss where a new physical therapy resident gets thrown in on orientation week and grilled by senior clinicians, this was probably how it would have unfolded.

I finished my questionable patient interview and proceeded with the physical exam. It was also a mess. I forgot to put on gloves when touching a steri-stripped surgical wound, measured the post-operative joint line inaccurately, and constantly had the patient cutting me off to jump in and give me feedback on how to do my evaluation. With Chris jumping in to also give feedback, the combined input was a bit much to say the least. On a positive note, at the end of the session, the patient said, "Good job, Kid," and gave me a high five. I took it for what it's worth and told myself it can only go up from here.

The first week ended, and with it came a short respite over the weekend to review my notes, gather my thoughts, and prepare to treat patients independently. As I would learn the hard way, all of my preparation over the weekend was to be hilariously inadequate.

CHAPTER 2

Mentoring Introductions

Transitioning into a new role is always challenging. Challenges that I faced at the start of residency included the chaotic inheritance of patients I was unfamiliar with, cumbersome navigation of a new documentation system workflow, and the ever-present nature of modified work procedures secondary to working close to the frontlines in the middle of a global pandemic. I would be lying if I said residency had a smooth start. I did not feel as if I knew what I was doing, and many times patients could tell that I was new. Some gave me a chance. Others never came back.

In the residency, the program had something called "Mentoring Time." The year was split into 3 trimesters, with an assigned mentor for each trimester. Once a week, my assigned mentor and I would meet. My mentor would observe me treating patients, and then we would discuss patient cases. Mentoring time was the most stressful part of the week, but also the most rewarding. At the end of each trimester, the resident would switch from one mentor to the next mentor.

I met my first mentor, Harvey, during my second week of residency. Tall, gregarious, and passionate about plants, he was quite the character to have for mentoring sessions. Our first mentoring session featured introductions, expectations, and clinical insights for consideration interspersed with references to plants to satisfy his inner plant personae.

"You can think of the trimesters as each having a theme to them. The first trimester, we break the resident down. The second trimester, we break down the residents even more, and this puts residents in an interesting space of uncertainty. We start to build back up when we get to the third trimester, and then by the end of the residency, that's where it all comes back together."

As I went through residency, I found that each trimester did in fact have its own theme, individualized based on the needs of the resident and the strengths of the mentors. For my first trimester, one of the major themes was refining my skills with the patient interview, or as we call it in the physical therapy world, the subjective. The patient interview fascinated Harvey. Harvey's take was that while one could over the course of time consistently improve their physical exam skills, treatment techniques and exercise prescription, the subjective was always so variable. A physical therapist could certainly work on their ability to ask questions in various ways to obtain information, but the quality of the subjective also depended on the patient's ability to understand and answer the questions without excessive or unnecessary information. An excellent historian would typically make the encounter smoother, while a poor historian would lead to the necessity for more time spent asking questions or ultimately limited useful information. A patient who was easily distracted and went on tangents could potentially de-rail a conversation, spending more time on their first visit talking about their three cats and favorite TV show than the actual reason for why they were coming to physical therapy. While this could be a source of entertainment, visits have a finite amount of time and therefore the tangents cannot travel too far if the physical therapist hopes to obtain sufficient information to medically treat the patient.

As a plant aficionado, Harvey drew parallels between the refinement of patient interviewing skills and the art of growing bonsai trees.

> "There's this master bonsai tree grower in Japan who started his apprenticeship in his teenage years and did the apprenticeship for 11 years. He's regarded now as one of the best bonsai tree growers in the world. He's spent his entire life crafting these trees and now he's probably getting close to retiring. It's in a way similar to us working on our clinical expertise and the subjective. We spend our entire careers working to master it, and by the time we're at the height of our skill, we're right at the end of our careers before we retire…"

Mentoring with patient care the second week of residency started off in an unusual manner. On my very first evaluation during mentoring, my patient was referred to physical therapy for neck pain. This patient however had a very odd history, with long-term occasional headaches on one side of the head only reproduced semi-consistently with walking up hills. We were conducting the evaluation virtually on telehealth per our clinic's policy due to the pandemic, and after I finished asking all of the questions I could possibly think of, to try to determine possible reasons for his symptoms, I muted the microphone to chat with Harvey.

"So, what do you think is going on?" I sat in deep thought for what felt like an eternity, mentally running through all the possibilities for muscles, joints, nerves, ligaments, anything that could be contributing to this patient's suspiciously weird pain that seemed to not be neck related.

I conceded that I was clueless. "I have no idea." I held my breath for a second, waiting for Harvey to point out something critical, insightful, or obvious that I had missed or forgotten to ask about.

"I have no idea either." This almost felt like a pat on the back in my diagnostic experience in residency up till now. Harvey was equally stumped. Clearly, we were not dealing with something typical to the realm of orthopedic physical therapy.

After further discussion, evaluation, and a subsequent follow-up visit, it was determined that physical therapy was not the right place due to the patient's likely non-neuromusculoskeletal cause for their symptoms.

Over the course of the month, Harvey would observe me treating patients on a weekly basis, and he would occasionally contribute as needed during sessions. The bulk of our discussion would then occur after the patient care. Mentoring during the third week with Harvey was an eye-opener. I had a patient for a follow-up visit related to post-surgery shoulder rehabilitation. I ended up prescribing an active assisted range of motion exercise to move them in different directions and provide some basic strengthening. I thought the follow-up was very straightforward. Harvey thought otherwise.

Harvey proceeded to dissect this follow-up more than I did. He referenced the questions I could have asked about specific activities of daily living, advised to incorporate more creativity with the exercises I give, and inquired about integrating some active range of motion components into traditionally active assisted range of motion exercises with consideration for the glenohumeral joint's structure. The overarching theme? Be creative with how I think about clinical practice. "You don't want to be stuck in the same patterns doing the same thing 20 years from now." Duly noted. It was a good reminder to not get too comfortable at any point over the next year.

Getting too comfortable did not seem like it would be an issue in September, however. I proceeded to go through a series of other complicated patients. One patient presented at their evaluation with symptoms of progressively worsening back pain, worsening numbness and tingling in their legs, worsening bowel and bladder function, and progressively increasing difficulty with walking. These symptoms lined up very consistently with an emergency condition known as Cauda Equina syndrome, but I later found out that this patient ended up having those symptoms due to methamphetamine withdrawal. Another patient intentionally refused to give me straight answers during our encounters out of spite for "the system." Another patient aggressively questioned my ability to perform my job every visit simply because of how young I looked. Another patient during a video evaluation referred to physical therapy for back pain had a non-functioning camera, required a translator, and ended up being referred back to their primary care physician for high suspicion of undiagnosed end-stage cancer. All these challenges kept me on my toes, but I felt like I couldn't relax for a second when working in order to bring my best self to each workday.

At the end of the first month, Harvey and I were discussing the closure of my first month of residency and he came across the topic of the complexity of my patients. "That patient with Cauda Equina syndrome- like symptoms, I get like two patients in like 10 years with that." In contrast to Harvey's experience, I had already seen multiple patients requiring advanced medical screening and subsequent referral out to another provider at an average rate of once per week. "Cathy and I were talking, and you have a lot of really challenging patients. You have one of the most challenging starts I've ever seen for a resident or anyone starting a new job in general." I appreciated Harvey's ability to show me the big umbrella here as it was so easy to fall into the stressful coping of just getting through multiple complex evaluations.

I will admit, this first month of residency was quite a bit. There were a lot of challenging scenarios that I had to navigate, but reflecting back now on that start, I see there were many valuable insights that I gained. I have carried these over into my current practice since, and they continue to be useful to me. The challenges were far from over though. Residency would only get more challenging from here.

CHAPTER 3

The World of Telehealth

In early 2020, during my final year of school, I encountered telehealth for the first time. By March of that year, the California hospital system where I was treating patients had swiftly shifted to telehealth as a response to the COVID-19 pandemic, aiming to continue to deliver care while minimizing direct in-person contact. Fortunately, my location facilitated a relatively smooth and rapid transition, completing this shift in less than two weeks. To support clinicians in adapting, a 4-hour long, self-paced educational course covering the fundamentals of telehealth physical therapy examination and treatment was provided. Additionally, clear instructions for carrying out standardized procedures during telehealth visits were created and provided system-wide, ensuring a cohesive and effective implementation overall.

Through that rotation, I discovered both the wonderful positive side of telehealth and the chaotic, disorganized side of telehealth. In short, telehealth physical therapy involves the provision of physical therapy services through a video platform. The patient and therapist go through evaluation or treatment through video for the duration of the encounter, and the therapist treats mainly through a combination of exercise prescription and education.

Telehealth physical therapy care provided an interesting new dynamic to how clinical encounters could unfold. Ideally, both clinicians and patients log on from either a mostly isolated quiet space or log on from their homes. When people log on from their homes and must use their video cameras, each person can get insight into the other person's personal life. This insight can lead to laughs, awkward moments, connections, cameo appearances from babies and pets, and more shared between a patient and a physical therapist. As I have learned in my time doing telehealth physical therapy, cats are especially notorious for choosing intentionally to sit in front of the camera and obscure both my view of the patient and the patient's view of the computer screen. As the pandemic continued to progress into the Fall of 2020, residency became an opportunity to dive back once again into the world of telehealth care and the memorable aspects associated with it.

October-November 2020

A few notable telehealth encounters stick out in memory during these months, both during mentoring sessions and outside of mentoring sessions.

One patient during mentoring was evaluated for post-surgical care of her knee. The type of surgery itself and post-operative recovery thus far based on the medical chart review were relatively straightforward. Just about everything else in the encounter was more chaotic.

Harvey and I went into a treatment room to conduct the telehealth evaluation with the patient calling in virtually from her home. Less than a minute into the hour-long encounter, the internet on the patient's side started to cut out, and the audio feedback began to lag. Eventually, the internet connection was re-established, but for the duration of the hour, the internet was spotty. This forced me to repeat questions multiple times, burning precious time that should be used otherwise—to provide treatment for the patient.

The patient also only had her iPhone for conducting the video visit, which limited her options for camera positioning. This combined with her physical limitations related to her surgical repair made camera positioning particularly challenging. All attempts to position the camera by herself resulted in crystal clear views of the waist and zero visibility of the knee that I needed to assess. After multiple failed attempts at camera positioning, the patient conceded that she needed help.

> "Hang on, let me get my son… ROBERRTTT!!! GET OVER HERE AND HELP ME WITH THE CAMERA!!!"

It was clear to Harvey and me that this patient was very mad at her son. Her son came over to help with the camera positioning, and we finally had some half decent visualization of the knee.

Slightly further into this same patient encounter, the son left the room the patient was in, and the patient needed her son's help again with camera positioning.

> "ROBERRRTTT!!! GET BACK OVER HERE!!! I DIDN'T SAY YOU COULD LEAVE THE ROOM!!"

> "MA, I'M BUSY, WHY DO YOU NEED MY HELP STILL!?!?"

> "I'M NOT DONE YET WITH MY PHYSICAL THERAPY; NOW GET OVER HERE AND HOLD THE CAMERA!!"

The son came back into my patient's room and proceeded to argue intensely with the patient. Harvey and I sat in the treatment room, awkwardly staring at the computer as we waited for the argument to calm down. If there were a time to be grateful for the existence of the "Mute" button on Zoom and a face mask to cover my facial expression, this was certainly one of many times. We eventually finished the evaluation, and I made the decision to schedule the patient to come in person for follow-up care to try to avoid any more chaotic telehealth visits with her. All subsequent follow-up in-person visits with this patient were decidedly less chaotic.

∽

Another memorable telehealth patient encounter occurred for a patient not much older than I was at the time. We only had 3 encounters altogether, two over telehealth and one in person. Despite only a handful of interactions, each one had clear, notable aspects.

This patient was referred to physical therapy after they previously crashed while biking, hit their head on the ground, and had their bike hit their head. At the time, no imaging was done, but they went to the ER a couple weeks after due to a sudden significant increase in low back pain. No imaging for the neck was done there either, but imaging was done for the low back with no significant findings. Our first encounter was an evaluation over telehealth, and I was proceeding through my interview of the patient to get an understanding of their overall background and symptoms.

> "Can you tell me what kind of symptoms you're experiencing currently?"

> "Well, I have trouble lifting my hands over my head, and I can barely hold a smoothie or a 1 lb. weight. I keep having headaches and I keep having trouble with remembering things."

This patient proceeded to list a few other symptoms consistent with potential spinal cord damage secondary to trauma. Some alarm bells were going off in my head; this did not sound good in the slightest bit. Considering their history of traumatic injury to the neck and head, and lack of imaging on the neck to rule out any emergency conditions, thoughts started to race through my head as I tried to decide whether to tell them to go to the emergency room to get checked again or not. Should I tell them to go? Should I ask more questions? Half of the physical examination measures that I would have used for this exam at the time to determine if the patient needed to go or not couldn't be done because we were working virtually.

> "Can you tell me if your symptoms have been getting worse, getting better, or staying about the same?"

> "I don't really know, I think it's been getting worse, and I don't know what to do about it. I don't know if this is related to anything either, but I used to hit my head against the wall as a form of self-harm, and there were multiple times that I would do this." The patient started to become more frantic over the computer. "Do you think **that** has anything to do with my symptoms!?"

More alarm bells started going off in my head. Now, I had to not only determine if my patient needed to go to the emergency room or not, but I also needed to check on the patient to make sure they were not continuing to self-harm. I needed to gather more information and do so in way that did not create further anxiety and stress in this patient.

After some additional line of careful questioning, I was able to determine that the patient was no longer self-harming anymore, and that the self-harm era of life for them was years ago long before their recent bike injury. I was also able to determine that the patient did not yet need to go to the ER, but I advised the patient on symptoms to look out for just in case.

> "Have you ever discussed this self-harm history with another healthcare provider or checked with a healthcare provider about your neck?"

> "I haven't. You're the first one that's ever asked in detail about both of those things."

We continued to discuss her overall case, proceeded through a physical examination, and reviewed a treatment plan. We reached the end of our session with only a couple minutes left for the allotted time.

> "Do you have any last questions for me?"

> "I think I'm good for now, but thank you so much for the information, I really appreciated you checking in on my neck and on my overall health."

The patient logged off. I logged off as well, closed my computer, and pondered for a moment about the encounter. It seemed to me that this patient had been through a lot, and review of their medical chart indicated that there were a lot of other health related challenges going on in their life.

Follow-up visits were only allotted 30 minutes at my clinic. At my second encounter with this patient, the same patient was not logged in right on time. I waited to see if they would show up. It wasn't until 10 minutes later the patient finally logged on.

"I'm so sorry I'm late, I'm really going through a lot right now!" The patient began to sob uncontrollably. "My partner and I literally just broke up 20 minutes ago, and I don't know what I'm going to do, and I'm supposed to move out of my apartment this week and I don't know where to put all of my stuff!"

The patient continued to sob even more as I tried to console them, which took another 10 minutes. I had my lunch break scheduled right after, so I ended up taking extra time to go through the visit and answer questions, console the patient, and develop a plan for the patient's next visit. We agreed upon scheduling for a third visit in person, with this visit possibly being the last one due to their life circumstances of possibly moving out of state. We ended the call 20 minutes after the allotted time. As the call ended, I felt a wave of fatigue wash over me. I couldn't help but feel drained from all of the effort needed to stay present and supportive for this patient. Did I not care enough? Did I care too much? Honestly, I wasn't sure. Some days, I felt like 30 minutes wasn't enough time to successfully support a patient in their care, especially when other facets of their lives were seemingly collapsing around them.

Our third visit together was during a mentoring session. This patient came in, and I checked in on their symptoms. They reported that overall, they were doing more physical activity, had less pain, and could get their pain to calm down more easily. However, they seemed even more stressed and anxious than in their previous two encounters combined, and this showed in the sustained streams of questions and uncertainties that dominated our conversation:

"How do I know my pain is going to get better? I feel like my pain is never going to get better, and I feel like I need it to get better because I need to start exercising again because I've just gained so much weight over the last year and I feel like I've gained so much fat over the year and I NEED to trim the fat down as soon as possible because I feel really tired and lethargic. Like, what should I do for my nutrition plan? What's the best possible nutrition plan so that I can trim my fat down as fast as possible? Like how many carbs should I be eating, how much protein should I be eating, and is there a best ratio for the amount of fat that I should be taking in? What should I do for the best possible exercises to burn fat? How do I know the exercises I have now are going to get me better? I feel like just seeing you for only 30 minutes just isn't enough and I feel like I need to be seen more often, and would it be possible to see you 2 times a week? Or would it be possible if you could find someone for me in the place where I'm going to move to? Like I just don't know what my options are or what to do?"

I felt rather overwhelmed by the sheer volume of questions being unloaded. How many of them do I answer? Why were there so many? Where do I even start? I didn't really know how to answer everything without sitting for the next hour plus explaining things in full detail and felt obligated to maintain a strict timeline for the visit since this was a visit during a mentoring session with Harvey. I also had another patient scheduled right after this patient, so I ended up trying to choose my answers in a way that covered overarching themes for guidelines of gradual, safe return to exercise. I also advised the patient to consider consulting with a nutritionist if they felt that this would be helpful, and after a couple of changes to their exercise program, the visit concluded.

Although my next patient was arriving in person, there were similar themes to the previous patient of very heightened anxiety that was brought with them. This next patient had long term numbness and tingling in one of their arms that started only when the pandemic started, and they were forced to shift to working 15 to 16-hour days on the computer. Despite my best efforts to reassure this patient of our treatment plan, the patient still expressed a lot of anxiety and stress regarding their pain. It was a tough situation for this patient as their excessive work hours were likely a contributor for their symptoms, yet they didn't really have the option to make changes to their routine in order to give their body a chance to recover from daily fatigue and possible overuse issues that were mounting.

One week after those two patient encounters at our next mentoring session, Harvey and I were discussing how my mentoring as a whole was going. We were now in the heart of the Fall, well into the endeavors of residency.

"How do you think residency's going for you so far?"

I took a moment to ponder the question.

"Well, I think I'm getting faster with pulling information together to come to a primary diagnosis along with alternate diagnoses to consider, and I'm getting better at matching my interventions with my primary diagnosis. I think there's still room to grow though in being firm with patients and setting boundaries, and there's probably some room for redirecting conversations."

"I agree with you, I think we're thinking on the same page overall," Harvey nodded in agreement as he spoke. He continued, "One thing I want to remind you of is, don't forget to have fun with the process."

I was surprised by this piece of advice. Harvey said he was just as surprised at himself that he was giving this piece of advice.

"Usually, we're really trying to push the residents to their very limits. We keep pushing and pushing and pushing, and sometimes that can be a lot for the residents. I've been thinking about this, and both you and Mariano are laid back with residency and taking it well. There's a lot of people I think though that are coming to you with a lot of anxiety. Our last mentoring session, you had two people back-to-back, both with lots of anxiety, and I think part of that is the world that we live in now."

I nodded as I recalled the two patients from the previous week, and reflected upon their anxiety in the context of the current state of the world that we lived in. We lived in a world where a pandemic had taken almost 250,000 lives in the US at this point in November.[10] It was one that had induced poor work-life balance for many people including many of my patients, and it had taken a toll on this country both physically and mentally. Many times, patients brought stress, anxiety, and tears with them to the clinic, and while I tried as best as I could to help them, sometimes I felt like I couldn't.

Often, I found myself asking: "To what extent do I as a physical therapist support patients with needs outside of what's written on the referral?" I would continue to ask myself this question throughout residency. Even after residency, I continue to keep asking myself that question and to reflect on it.

CHAPTER 4

Introducing Students to Clinical Practice

OCTOBER – NOVEMBER 2020

By mid-Fall, our residency routine was well established. Mariano and I were occupied 5 days a week taking care of patients, attending advanced clinical education courses, and helping to teach in the physical therapy program that we had freshly graduated from. Although our scheduled responsibilities amounted to about 40 hours per week on paper, the reality of residency was that we were spending much more time than that on residency related work. At least once per week, I found myself staying after working hours in the clinic with Mariano, practicing hands-on treatment techniques or discussing upcoming assignments related to our teaching responsibilities or monthly journal club. Weekends were often spent reading countless pages of research articles related to the classes we were taking, trying to keep up with research related to the latest advances in physical therapy.

As part of the residency, Mariano and I also had the opportunity to serve as clinical instructors for first-year physical therapy students. Each of us was supervising students who were stepping into the clinic for two days before going back into the classroom. This was my first chance to mentor students in a clinical setting, and I can firmly say that I enjoyed the overall experience. A couple of patient encounters stick out in memory from my time with my students.

When I looked at my schedule of patients for Day 1 with my first set of students, to my surprise, I saw the residency-trained physical therapist that I had evaluated for Chris at the beginning of residency on my schedule. Turns out Chris needed them to be seen for care for one visit before going back to him with his schedule being full. Once in a while, patients who were primarily seeing one PT would end up seeing another PT in the interim based on medical necessity, and in this case, it was warranted. I suspected that my first-year students were going to be just as thrown off, if not more thrown off than I was, meeting this patient for the first time. This was going to be entertaining.

In the morning, I met with my students. We did introductions, discussed expectations, reviewed the charts for the patients, and then got to work in the clinic. Late morning, the patient came to the clinic. We exchanged pleasantries and then started to make our way to a treatment table where my students were waiting.

"So, I have a couple students with me today. Are you okay with them observing and possibly helping with treatment?"

"You have students!? How the *fuck* do *you* have students already!?" Clearly my patient was surprised. "You're only two months in and you already have students?" (For context, it is uncommon in the physical therapy profession as a whole for someone who's been practicing for less than 3 months to be doing any kind of supervision for students).

INTRODUCING STUDENTS TO CLINICAL PRACTICE

Fortunately, the patient was more than happy to have my students around for the visit and proceeded to dole out plenty of feedback for my students regarding their measuring technique, handling skills and exercise selection. The students were a little unsure of how to handle my patient's high energy and lack of filter, but nevertheless navigated the encounter successfully with a couple crisp high fives to end the visit.

On Day 2 with the same students, I had a follow-up with one of my patients who I had been seeing since the start of residency for shoulder surgery rehabilitation. He missed his appointment the day before because he was meant to log on to Zoom but failed to do so during his allotted 30-minute appointment slot on my schedule. On this day with my students, he remembered to log in on time. Typically, the first words from a patient doing a telehealth visit were confirmation of their full name, location, and verbal consent for treatment. Today, this was not the case.

"Dude, I'm so sorry man, I spaced out yesterday and I was pretty fucking pissed at myself for missing it. I was checked in, and then I spaced out for a sec, and then it was past the time, and I was like 'Fuck!'"

My students and I got a laugh out of that. I wasn't particularly concerned that he missed the visit the day before as long as he was able to make it to this visit and as long as he was overall doing okay. The rest of the visit went by smoothly and we were able to get the next visit set up. On a positive note, this patient didn't miss any more of his visits for the duration of time that I treated him, and we overall got along well.

As I watched my first-year students perform patient interviews, teach exercises, and take measurements, I thought about how far I had come in my clinical practice. I could still remember distinctly when I was in my first year of school, I struggled so immensely with basic skills and speaking with people. Speaking with people for me as a first-year student was an especially daunting experience. As a resident, I still experienced times when I found myself feeling awkward while talking to a patient, but my comfort level overall had improved significantly. I also did not have to think as hard about how to do basic skills such as measuring range of motion, although I was now instead having to think really hard about higher level reasoning as a resident. I had certainly grown a lot, but still had a long way to go.

CHAPTER 5

The Ripple Effect of Politics

November 2020

Every four years in the United States, the election for the president occurs. This year was an election year, with the two main candidates being the then-current President Donald Trump facing off against former Vice President Joe Biden. In the clinic and amongst my patients, there was a sense of heightened anxiety and tension building as election day slowly creeped up.

Since the beginning of the COVID-19 pandemic in March 2020, I believed that the US's national-level response to the pandemic had been frustratingly lackluster. In past times of crisis such as during the World Wars in the 20th century, global crises served as a catalyst for uniting the country together. This pandemic was another opportunity for the country to come together once more and to work together, yet the political rhetoric that echoed across the country served mostly to divide the country and delay proper response to a highly infectious novel disease whose long-term effects are not understood as yet.

Compared to 2019, the rate of reported hate crimes against various people based on race, ethnicity and ancestry also increased significantly in 2020. My parents and I would have regular discussions about the rates of reported hate crimes against Asian Americans, which had almost doubled in 2020.[11] With my parents being first generation Taiwanese American immigrants and myself being a second-generation Taiwanese American, it was not lost on us that we could all be potential targets.

I recall one particular conversation with an older patient who was a first-generation immigrant from China. I worked with them through a Cantonese interpreter through a series of sessions and had established a good working dynamic. One day after the end of a session, I was working on scheduling them for their next visit.

> "Can you come to your next visit at 4:30 PM?" The interpreter relayed the question to the patient.

> The patient discussed briefly with the interpreter, and the interpreter replied, "They cannot come at that time, because they have to take the bus across the city, and they don't feel safe if it's too late."

The translation from the interpreter, combined with the patient's tone and brief look of apprehension gave me a moment's pause. It made me think about how hateful rhetoric directed at Asians and Asian Americans had been echoed throughout the year in the US. It made me think about Donald Trump's rhetoric back in the Summer, when he referred to COVID-19 as "Kung Flu." It made me think about how my parents worried about me not only because I was in healthcare and at increased risk of exposure to COVID-19, but also because I sometimes had to stay late at night in the clinic which to my parents was a potentially unsafe thing to do. As I chose an alternate preferred time for the patient and printed out their handout for their exercises, I looked at my patient and thought about how this patient could be someone's parent, someone's grandparent, someone's beloved family member. I walked to the printer to pick up the printout, reflecting about how I wished for a world where people could just ride the bus at any time of the day without worrying about having a hate crime committed against them. I handed the printout to the patient and told them that I'll see them next time and to reach out if there were any questions. The patient thanked me and as they departed, I thought about how hard living with the pandemic has been, and I told my patient as they left that I looked forward to our next meeting.

This particular patient encounter was just one instance of reflecting on the ripple effect of racism and politics, how both can have the far-reaching impact of influencing a person's day-to-day routine and creating barriers to healthcare access. As a healthcare provider, I will always advocate for ways to reduce the barriers for healthcare access and encourage every other provider who reads this book to do the same. If that means trying extra hard to schedule accessible times for patients, working little by little to dismantle personal implicit biases or advocating for concrete action to dismantle systemic racism, then so be it. It is hard work, but work that is worth doing is seldom easy.

Perhaps in a different life stage, there would be further concrete action I could take to be an advocate for equitable care. Residency and its challenges would continue to proceed though, impartial to the struggles of Asian American immigrants seeking care and healthcare providers trying to provide said care.

December 2020

The end of the first trimester of residency was approaching and we had entered the winter. I was working with a patient who I had been seeing for some time now for a few different diagnoses. This patient and I had built a good working relationship, and we enjoyed discussing a myriad of topics during consultations. One morning, I logged on to my computer and set up Zoom to wait for the patient. The patient logged in on time as usual, and after verifying consent for treatment, we began the session.

"How are you feeling overall since I last saw you?"

"Well, I have some questions about a few things, but let me tell you this: I don't know what it is, I've just been feeling kind of down for the last few weeks because of all the things that have been happening in the world, and I've never been diagnosed with depression before or anything like that. I just want to check with you, is it normal to feel what I'm feeling? Does this kind of stuff have an effect on how my body feels pain?"

This patient had been thinking a lot over the last few weeks about the cumulative toll of the pandemic, changes to their personal life due to the pandemic, and the election. We discussed the relationship between stress and the body's perception of pain. We then talked some more regarding their care.

Once the patient's questions were answered, the patient thanked me, logged off, and the visit ended. The impression on me didn't end though, but rather stuck with me for the rest of the day. This patient was not the first to express these types of sentiments to me. Many others before them had expressed similar sentiments of feeling anxious, tired, stressed, and saddened. It was a reminder that this work has its share of heavy moments, and the pandemic wasn't making it any easier. Our meeting was also a reminder that I would have to help ease people's anxieties, fears, and stresses, and provide them reassurance that things will be okay in the end, even as I too carried some of these stresses and anxieties with me through this uncertain time.

During December 2020, the United States as a whole continued to struggle with managing the pandemic, a product in my mind of the failure at the national government level to unify the country combined with resultant mistrust in the doctors and scientists who specialize in infectious diseases. The US had crossed 300,000 deaths due to COVID-19 and was currently at over 16 million reported cases.[12] The FDA had done emergency authorization of a COVID-19 vaccine from Pfizer, and my clinic site sent out emails announcing plans for the upcoming vaccine distribution. In my journal for this week, I wrote a note at the end:

> "I continue to pray that I can keep myself and my family safe. I'm so close to getting the first round of the vaccine. It would be especially heartbreaking to get infected now, bring it back to my parents, and get them infected."

CHAPTER 6

The First Live Patient Examination (LPE)

In residency, there were a series of examinations in order to test the knowledge and skills of the residents. There were 3 types of examinations. The first was technique practical examinations (two in the year) assessing a resident's ability to perform advanced treatment and assessment techniques with appropriate rationale. The second was written examinations (two in the year) for testing our clinical foundational knowledge. Finally, the third type of examination was what each trimester concluded with, an examination called the Live Patient Examination, or LPE.

The LPE is perhaps the most challenging and most unpredictable of the examinations. Under the supervision of 2 proctors, I was to perform a 60-minute evaluation on a real patient, including a patient interview, physical exam, and treatment. After the patient interview, my proctors and I were to step off to the side to discuss my thought process for a ranked order of the three most likely anatomical contributors to their symptoms and rationale to accompany my choices (The choices on this list will be referred to interchangeably as my diagnoses and hypotheses). After performing the physical exam, my proctors and I were to step off to the side again to discuss any changes to my initially generated top three list and rationale to accompany the new list before going into treatment. After completing the visit with treatment, I was given 45 minutes to complete both my documentation on the patient evaluation, and a reflection form to prepare for an oral defense. After 45 minutes, I would then perform an oral defense where the proctors would grill me on my clinical reasoning, critiquing my rationale for why I made my choices and whether my rationale for my choices was sound or not.

The element of evaluating a real patient adds a layer of uncertainty to the clinical encounter. Because patients are people and because people are unique, no two live patient examinations are alike. My experience with all of my live patient examinations was that none of them were simple or straightforward, and my first LPE was very memorable on multiple levels.

December 2020

Prior to my first LPE, I was allowed to see the patient on my schedule and could review their chart. The chart review unfortunately did not tell me much info other than that they were being referred in for "neck and shoulder pain," and that they were interested in physical therapy. I reviewed all of my notes from classes, created diagnosis lists, and reviewed possible treatment options for this patient.

The day of the LPE arrived, and I went to the clinic. My proctors are my current mentor Harvey and my upcoming subsequent mentor, Kenny. While waiting for the patient, I chatted with the two of them, keeping an eye on my computer to see when my patient would check in. I felt surprisingly calm, as I did not really know what to expect with the whole LPE experience. I also provided my initial diagnosis list for consideration, which in hindsight was a pretty garbage diagnosis list due to the multiple assumptions I was making with the limited information I had. I was counting heavily on getting more concrete information after interviewing my patient in order to make my diagnosis list stronger, which historically for me had not been too much of an issue until now. When my computer showed me that the patient had checked in, I walked over to the lobby to get my patient. It was Go Time.

I called out my patient's name, and my patient walked over. The overall appearance was not what I was expecting. My patient had super long, unkempt hair that was possibly greasy. Complementing the hair was a pungent body odor that smelled of pasta sauce mixed with sweat. To cap it off, an air of social awkwardness seemed to permeate my patient. This was a very, very different patient from all of my other patients ever experienced until now. Still, I wasn't panicking quite yet.

I led the patient to the back treatment table that we were using for the LPE, introduced myself, and began asking questions for my patient interview.

"Can you point to where exactly you have pain?"

"Well, it's kind of hard to pinpoint, but I kind of get it here, and sometimes I get it here, and sometimes I get it over here."

My patient drew large circles with their hand around the area of their right neck and right shoulder region, circles that were large enough that they didn't really help me narrow down to specific parts of the body that could be used to improve the precision of my diagnosis list.

I started to point to specific points on the neck and shoulder region.

THE FIRST LIVE PATIENT EXAMINATION (LPE)

"Would you say around the center of here?" "Well, I mean maybe." "Okay, what about this part of your neck?" "Well maybe, it's hard to say."

What should have usually taken less than 30 seconds for a patient who was a half decent historian had already taken about 5 minutes due to the need for clarification. Time was of the essence, and I knew that I needed to be more efficient in obtaining information. I was starting to sweat a little bit.

"Can you tell me what makes your pain worse?" "Well, I don't really know."

"Can you tell me when you get pain?" "I don't really know that."

"What about looking up at the ceiling?" "Well, I don't really know."

"Okay, what about looking down at the ground?" "Well, I'm unsure."

"What about turning your head to look around?" "Well, it's hard to say."

"Okay, what about going to pick up a heavy object off the ground?" "Well, I would never do that, so I don't know."

"What about reaching to unlock a car door?" "Uh, it's hard to say."

"What about reaching behind your back?" "I mean, maybe, I don't know."

"Well, is there anything you can think of that makes your pain worse?" "Well, the weather makes it worse."

"Is there anything besides the weather that makes your pain worse?" "It's hard to say, I'm not sure."

Panic mode was starting to rapidly sink in. I was no closer to gathering anything vaguely useful to me for changing my diagnosis list. I changed strategies and moved away from trying to figure out a specific pain reproducing action.

"Can you tell me what kinds of things make your pain better?" "Well, my partner does this massage thing that kind of hurts and then that kind of makes it feel better."

"Is there anything else that you can think of that makes your pain better?" "I mean, not really."

"Does rest help your pain?" "I think that helps, but it's hard to say."

Panic mode was continuing to escalate rapidly, and I was sweating even more. Perhaps asking about the things they had trouble with doing in their daily life would give me some insight.

"Can you tell me what kinds of things in your daily life you're not able to do because of your pain?" "Well, I can do everything I need to do."

THE FIRST LIVE PATIENT EXAMINATION (LPE)

"What about anything related to your work?" "Well, I work in IT and once in a while I have pain with using a computer and mouse."

Usually by this point of the patient interview, I would have used about 15 minutes to talk with the patient, and I would have had a half decent idea of what I wanted to establish for my possible diagnosis list. Instead, I was already at over 20 minutes of the allotted 60 minutes and had no idea what I was going to do or what I was going to say to my proctors. Panic mode was cranked up to the max. There was a healthy portion of internal screaming occurring. I felt the armpits of my shirt becoming soaked from my profuse sweating.

My proctors and I stepped into a separate treatment room to discuss my hypothesis list. I gave my unchanged, highly questionable diagnosis list and the best possible rationale that I could come up with. I knew that the rationale I provided was also highly questionable, and it was pretty obvious to my proctors that I had no idea what some of the plausible anatomical structures contributing to this patient's pain were. My proctors told me after the testing portion of the LPE that they were really, really worried that I wasn't going to pass this LPE.

I transitioned to the physical exam. I was nervous. Very nervous. I knew that I was going to be very heavily dependent on my physical exam to give me something tangible to work with for a diagnosis. I proceeded through my range of motion and strength testing for the neck and for the shoulder. I was searching for something, anything that would reproduce either my patient's neck pain or the shoulder pain. My physical exam also took almost 20 minutes as I continued to search and search and search.

I had the patient lie face-down so I could perform my final assessment technique on the neck. This was my last hope. If I found nothing here, I was probably doomed to fail. I carefully worked through assessing each portion of the patient's neck.

"How does this part of your neck feel?" "Uh, it feels okay."

"How about this part?" "Uh, that feels fine too."

"How about here?" "Uh, that hurts." "Okay, where does it hurt?" "It hurts in my neck and my shoulder."

In the chaotic storm of half-baked clinical reasoning and stress clouding my mind, a light of clarity shined through. I found something tangible that reproduced the patient's symptoms! I had less than 20 minutes left. At that moment, I knew this was my only chance to try to provide meaningful treatment to the patient and give myself a chance to pass the LPE. I threw out my entire original plan, pivoted towards this piece of information, and fully committed to treatment based on this one piece of information. I picked a treatment technique to address the mobility of this patient's neck, performed it, and re-assessed their range of motion. Their range of motion improved!

"How do you feel?" "Well, I think I feel a little better."

It seemed to be working! I had limited time left so I provided a couple exercises aimed at mimicking my treatment technique, scheduled the patient for their follow-up visit, and then concluded the evaluation.

I didn't have any time to document during the evaluation, so the bulk of the 45 minutes afterwards was spent trying to rip through completing documentation as fast as possible while also working on the reflection form in conjunction. After my allotted documen-

THE FIRST LIVE PATIENT EXAMINATION (LPE)

tation and reflection time concluded, I met with the two proctors to discuss the case.

"So, what are your initial thoughts for this case?"

I pondered the question and gathered my thoughts. "I felt like it was really challenging to obtain information from the patient that would have helped me."

We proceeded through a series of questions examining my overall thought process, rationale for evaluation techniques, rationale for the treatment options I made, and whether I would do anything different or not. There were additional questions throughout to really go through the layers of my reasoning, and lots of gaps that could have been improved upon. Of all the things that I had experienced during the first trimester of residency, this LPE was the single biggest thing that really highlighted a lot of my shortcomings as a clinician. Both of my proctors told me that my not being able to give an anatomical list for hypotheses was a huge red flag of my questionable reasoning skills for both of them. With that said, both of them were really happy to see that I was able to pivot mid-evaluation, change my direction, and adapt with a stronger hypothesis that ultimately led me to better treatment and direction with care. I didn't know whether I had passed or not until I checked for my feedback form online later that week. In order to pass this LPE, I needed to score at least 70%. I ended up scoring exactly 70%, leaving no points to spare this time around. What an absolute rollercoaster that LPE had been.

One reflection I took away from this LPE was that in the next trimester, I really wanted to keep working on the types of questions I asked. A few categories included:

– What are good questions to ask to rule diagnoses as more likely or less likely contributors?

– What are good questions to get a particular answer while being efficient?

– How can I ask fewer questions throughout the consultation and spend more time listening to the patient?

I had discussed the art of asking questions with Harvey. He had talked about how questions with similar pieces of information could be spun in different ways, and these subtle differences could help direct a conversation in one way or another. I anticipated that this would be an interesting space to explore not just for the rest of residency, but for the remainder of my career.

With the LPE completed, there was still a written exam and a technique practical exam left to complete. Thankfully, neither of these were nearly as stressful as the LPE. The written exam was completed online while on a Zoom call with Alison and Mariano, and each of us could log off once we were finished. The technique practical exam involved demonstrating and discussing a few selected hands-on treatment techniques that we had learned throughout the trimester. For this portion, Harvey and Alison were the proctors. When I got done and after we had discussed overall feedback, they let me know that I had passed the first round of everything. Both of them emphatically congratulated me, anticipating some sort of reciprocal expression of happiness combined with relief. Instead, I just kind of sat, feeling deflated and exhausted.

I didn't feel accomplished or excited despite the fact that everything technically was on pace so far. I was still thinking about how hard I had tried on the LPE, and how my current clinical skillset was only just barely enough to enable me to scrape by. I was still

THE FIRST LIVE PATIENT EXAMINATION (LPE)

successful though, and I felt that I'd learned so much as a clinician in the previous few months. In the process though, I was starting to truly realize that there was so much more that I needed to learn.

CHAPTER 7

A Dark Winter Ahead

December 2020

As the end of the calendar year approached, the residents had scheduled time off around the holidays. Holidays were traditionally a time to go home during school, and in any other year would have been a time to go home and rest from residency without a second thought. As cases and deaths related to COVID-19 started to spike across the state and country, I remained uncertain as to whether I should stay at my apartment to isolate just in case or travel home an hour's drive away to see my family. On one hand, I was incredibly exhausted from the demands of residency and time with family would have been a much-needed respite. On the other hand, even though I had made many efforts to minimize my risk of exposure to COVID-19, the thought of last-minute exposure, becoming an asymptomatic carrier and exposing my family to this virus weighed heavily on me. Should I go home? Should I not? I didn't know what the right answer would be.

In one of our team meetings, one of our clinic supervisors informed us that my affiliated hospital system was starting to provide COVID-19 vaccinations in waves stratified by risk of exposure to COVID-19. Based on the risk stratification, physical therapists were in the second tier of the first group, which meant that I was

A DARK WINTER AHEAD

predicted to get the vaccine sometime in January. We were also warned that cases of the virus were expected to skyrocket over the winter and to continue to make efforts to mitigate risk as best as possible. My final journal entry for the first trimester of residency was written late December, and I wrote the following:

> As of this writing, we had over 200,000 new COVID-19 cases yesterday.[13] The US sits at 18.2 million cases, with 322,000 deaths.[14] The world as a whole is at 77.6 million cases, with 1.71 million deaths worldwide.[15] At times, I am disheartened by how much the US has struggled as a whole and how little support there seems to be for essential workers, a whole generation of students, or for small businesses. I still very vividly remember stories from the early days of the pandemic. Stories of healthcare workers suiting up in trash bags to treat patients because there wasn't enough PPE to go around. Stories of patients overwhelming the hospital systems. Stories of patients dying in the hallways of hospitals, away from loved ones, with nobody around except for strangers suited in protective gear.

> Despite the suffering that continues to unfold, there is hope. There is a light at the end of the dark tunnel that has been 2020. Both Moderna and Pfizer have received FDA approval for emergency use authorization, and the vaccines may become widely available to the public by this upcoming spring.[16,17] We are headed into a dark winter though. Cases have skyrocketed and I fear that they will continue to skyrocket with the holidays this year. I will continue to do my best with supporting the healthcare system, protecting myself and trying to protect my family.

With the conclusion of the first trimester of residency, I went on a scheduled break. There were many challenges already within the first few months. I anticipated that there would be many more to come. After a two-week break over the holidays, it was time to transition to the second trimester of residency and the second part of this year-long journey.

PART 2:

The Second Trimester

CHAPTER 8

New Year, New Learning Curve

The new calendar year had arrived, and with it the second trimester of residency. I was a little rusty in my clinical skills getting back into patient care, but with each day, I slowly got readjusted to treating patients. Mentoring sessions with Harvey were now concluded, and Harvey passed the mentoring torch on to my second mentor, Kenny. Kenny was someone I was already acquainted with through physical therapy school. Given our pre-established relationship, I placed a high degree of trust in Kenny as a mentor, to facilitate my growth knowing that he came from a good place, even if that meant giving some tough love with his feedback. Kenny brought a different dynamic to mentoring sessions as well with his prior work experience in a private practice clinic, which is a very different work environment from a hospital-affiliated clinic.

In a hospital affiliated setting, it can be very, very challenging to keep track of all of one's patients. There is also often a high demand for patients trying to get in for care. By the time I finished residency, patient care volumes were returning to close to pre-pandemic numbers and the average wait time to get in for an appointment was somewhere between 6 weeks and 2 months. Because of the constant influx of patient referrals, if a patient already in the system decided to stop coming back to PT for any reason, there would always be another patient to take their place. In contrast, not all private practice settings have a guaranteed high volume of referrals. This means that in order to keep patients coming to the clinic, unless the clinic resorts to unethical methods of getting patients to come or stay, therapists need to really focus on making sure they provide value to the patient and that the patient believes that the time and money spent is well justified. The skill of providing value to patients partially comes from refining the art of being able to closely connect with patients.

If I had to choose a theme for the second trimester (in addition to the further so-called "breakdown of the resident"), I would say that it was about cultivating my ability to connect with patients. Through this trimester, I reflected more intentionally about trying to work together actively and collaboratively with my patients to establish a sincere and ever-evolving connection. I had thought up to this point that I was already doing a somewhat decent job of trying to connect with my patients, but as I would soon find out during this trimester, there was still a significant amount of growing that I needed to undergo.

January 2021

Undeniably, this trimester started off action-packed. I was back in the clinic again treating patients. Coursework was also continuing to build. Our first two courses for the trimester were on the topic of treating the shoulder, and the clinical faculty teaching the courses assigned a total of 21 different research publications for us to read over a span of 2 weeks. I still have all of those publications for reference, and by my estimation, it amounted to a total of around 300 pages of dense research literature, plus a couple of pre-course assignments. Welcome Back to Residency!

I had my first mentoring session with my new mentor, Kenny. During this session, I was evaluating a patient over telehealth who was preparing to go into surgery in about 2 months' time. Our initial greetings went smoothly, the evaluation went relatively smoothly, and the treatment was appropriate. The patient had an overall very pleasant demeanor, and we were connecting well. I then proceeded to the scheduling portion of the visit. I was not as good at managing the sheer number of patients on my schedule as I should have been leading up to this patient encounter. When I looked, I found that my schedule was much fuller than I anticipated.

> "So, based on my schedule, I can schedule you for a visit at the end of the month, and then we could do another visit a few weeks after in late February."

> "Well, hang on a minute, if we just schedule those visits, and then I have my surgery this date, that means I'm only going to see you two times before I get surgery! What am I supposed to do with only two visits before surgery!?" The tone of the patient had flipped, and they were suddenly starting to get frustrated with me.

I tried to salvage the situation. "I hear you, but this is my current availability. I will try to get back to you later this week to see if there's another therapist that can also help." This was a poor choice of words for a few reasons:

- Whether intended or not, talking about my limited schedule availability projected that I prioritized the numbers management piece rather than the individual patient in front of me.

- The phrasing of "I hear you," followed by the scheduling conversation piece could be interpreted as, "I understand your concern but don't really care enough to make the effort to address said concern."

– My choice of words of "later this week" was vague and didn't relay confidence to the patient that I was going to get back to them in a timely manner.

The patient was starting to get even more frustrated with me. Kenny could sense much more keenly than I could that I was ruining this encounter, and jumped in. "We will do the best that we can to get you in for more visits to address your needs, and we will get back to you with an answer by this Thursday or Friday." The patient acknowledged Kenny's statement (as the adult in the room, which was somewhat humiliating), and thanked him. The visit encounter ended shortly thereafter, and I was supposed to have my next patient come to the clinic for a follow-up. The patient was late however, so Kenny and I had time to debrief the evaluation. Kenny said to me, "Let's go to a treatment room to talk." We walked over to a room. Kenny closed the door, and his demeanor changed in an instant. He elevated his voice to one that was mixed with stern harshness and disappointment.

"You lost the patient! You lost them! You were doing really well, and then you lost them with the scheduling! Right now, that patient probably feels like they're not being cared about with only two visits before surgery!"

I sat in my chair, stunned by his cutting critique of the encounter as I replayed it in my mind. At the time of the encounter, I could kind of tell that the patient was getting mad, but did I really mess up that badly?

"You need to figure out your scheduling, because you have a problem right now with it being as full as it is. If I were that patient, and you scheduled me with only two visits spaced so far apart like that, I would be *pissed*!"

"Well, our schedules are preset, and…" Kenny cut me off.

"Well, you need to take responsibility for your schedule!"

Kenny then pointed at me briefly to highlight his next questions:

"What kind of physical therapist do you want to be? Do you want to be someone that just gives the "standard of care?" Or, do you want to go above and beyond, and be the best possible therapist that you can be? Do you want to be the type of therapist who people ask to see?"

He let those questions hang in the air for a few moments as I absorbed it in and processed it. My goal of course was to become the best possible therapist that I could be. Kenny's critiques really forced me to re-examine my choice of words and actions during the encounter, as well as re-evaluate just how much more growth I needed to undergo to become proficient at making patients feel valued. One of the big themes I took away from this encounter is:

> Even if I truly care about a patient, that intent is worth nothing if I don't do a good job conveying that care through my actions and making the patient really feel that they are being genuinely valued.

Everything from body language to word choice, tone and more could all contribute to each conversation I had with my patients.

My ability to read both verbal and non-verbal signs would also contribute to my overall degree of success connecting with patients and successfully treating them.

I was silent for what seemed like an eternity. Kenny could tell from my body language that his feedback, although very much essential, was weighing heavily on me and eating at me. His tone softened as he continued:

> "Technically, what you did was not necessarily wrong from a clinic logistics standpoint. However, it was still not in the best interest of that patient. If I were you, I would consider a transfer of care to another therapist with more availability in their schedule as one option in order to get the patient the care they need, and I would call this patient before the end of tomorrow."

I attempted to make amends later that day to talk with one of the other therapists to get the patient on their schedule, and then called the patient the next day to speak with them. Ultimately though, I had lost this patient. As a healthcare provider, it can be easy to assume that when patients come to you, they'll automatically feel that you have their best interest at heart. An upcoming surgery would most likely be very much on this patient's mind during this visit; failure to meaningfully set up this patient for pre-operative success was perceived as attempting to provide healthcare without the "care" portion. I believe it is the onus of healthcare providers to make the effort to bring intentional care to their patients, to not only bring a *light* to their patients, but to also reflect diligently on how they can keep building the capacity of that light.

CHAPTER 9

Hope

Hope can come in many forms. It can come in spoken words, handwritten letters, or a thoughtful card. It could also be a gift basket, an announcement, or a motto. Hope can be conceptual, or it can take a physical form.

For the duration of my last clinical rotation for physical therapy school and the first few months of residency, I would go to the clinic to work with patients, trying my best to protect myself and to minimize my risk of contracting COVID-19. The risk of getting myself and my family sick was always in the back of my mind and would weigh on me from time to time. I was not keen on finding out what would happen if I did get COVID-19, nor was I keen on becoming the reason my parents got infected. Through all of this uncertain time, many of my colleagues and I wondered when a safe and effective vaccine would become available to us. All of us and our patients held on to a hope that the national response to the pandemic would improve, that news of people dying by the thousands wouldn't become the new norm. We all held on to the hope that life would one day get better, that light would dispel the dark.

January – February 2021

Outside of residency, the nation continued to be embroiled in the pandemic and political conflict. On January 6th, supporters of Donald Trump stormed The Capitol building and occupied the building for hours in an effort to throw out the results of this past November's election.[18] The attempt was not successful, although for a time in the clinic, there was a sense of heightened fear that something could happen again. The inauguration of President Joe Biden and Vice President Kamala Harris occurred later this month.[19]

I remember one patient distinctly around this time for both our mutual passion for running and for the snippets of conversation related to politics that would occur at each visit. During one of our visits right after the inauguration, I asked them if they had had a chance to watch.

> "Oh yes, I did Derek! It was wonderful! I didn't move from the couch for like two hours, and I just sat there crying while watching! And then I watched it again for another couple hours later that night!"

> The patient continued, "In the neighborhood I work in, normally people are rough, and nobody really smiles. For the first time in a long time in the neighborhood where I work, people seemed *sooo* happy! Like life was normal again!"

I reflected on this joyous expression from my patient and the scene from the neighborhood that they painted, a capsule of the feeling of hope that many of us including myself felt during this time. There was much struggle, chaos, division, and suffering to get this far in the pandemic. Although the overall outcome resulting from this transfer of presidency and the subsequent office term may have ended up differently from what some people had hoped for, at the time, the mood in the clinic amongst all the patients and staff was undeniable. It felt like we had a chance now. A chance to bring this pandemic to a quicker end. A chance to try once more to face the systemic issues stemming from racism. A chance to rebuild a light.

The news of COVID-19 vaccines becoming available represented another form of hope. For me, having myself fully vaccinated and my family fully vaccinated represented hope. By this time of the pandemic, two vaccines for COVID-19 had emergency use authorization approval: one from Pfizer, and one from Moderna.[20,21] Across the nation, many locations were struggling to distribute their vaccine shipments to their essential workers efficiently and effectively.[22] I was very fortunate that my affiliated hospital system was doing a stellar job with the distribution process.

I went to receive my first dose of the Moderna vaccine at the beginning of the year. I must admit, it felt a little surreal to get the vaccine in a time when less than 10% of the entire country had received the vaccine. At my vaccination site, as I was waiting in line, a staff member gave us instructions to wait after receiving the dose in case of side effects and to not take pictures for privacy reasons. After about 15 minutes of waiting outside, we were permitted to enter the vaccination site. The nurse asked for my name, confirmed my date of birth, asked if I had any questions, and then administered the vaccine.

I sat in my designated chair for another 15 minutes, self-monitoring for any side effects while reflecting on the significance of the moment. The world had changed so much since last Spring when the COVID-19 virus was first declared a global health emergency and images from the hospitals in New York and Italy flooded the news feeds. I thought about how many people had lost their lives and loved ones due to COVID-19. I thought about all the sacrifices made by essential workers, all the sleepless hours spent by scientists and researchers racing against the clock to develop safe and effective vaccines. I wondered about how many more deaths there would be. I wondered how much longer the pandemic would loom over life.

When I went to get my second dose of the Moderna vaccine a month later, a similar train of thoughts flowed through my mind. Accompanying the thoughts this time though was a sense of optimism. I felt hopeful at the time for the pandemic to reach a decisive end in the near future. I felt gratitude towards the countless fellow healthcare providers directly supporting the care of patients with COVID-19, as well as those who made the vaccines possible. I reaffirmed my personal promise to keep working hard in residency, to make sure that I could contribute even a small part of bringing patients comfort and reassurance in addition to treatment for healing of their various ailments and injuries. For me, the administration of the vaccine was a light being passed on to me, and I felt just a little more inspired to pay it forward, to pass some light on to my patients.

CHAPTER 10

Never a Dull Moment

As I have noted during the introduction of this book, healthcare is one of the great intersections of humanity. There were some more memorable interactions with patients during the Winter and the beginning of Spring that I recount. At this stage of residency, I was experiencing a mix of emotions with patient care. A couple of my patients whom I had been treating since the start of residency had dropped off of my schedule. One of them wanted to switch physical therapists as I was seemingly not able to provide the care that they needed. Another wanted to pursue other non-physical therapy options as their condition had not responded at all to everything I had tried and could possibly think of. A few more patients had fallen off of my schedule due to other medical complications, and a few others were "no shows" to their appointments. It was times like this that would leave me questioning myself and wondering if there was more that I could do, more that I was missing.

February – March 2021

There was never a dull moment during mentoring. There were only interesting moments, extra interesting moments, and memorable moments. During one of my mentoring sessions with Kenny, another clinical faculty member joined for our session to observe as well as to give additional feedback on top of what Kenny provided. I distinctly remember the patient I was evaluating for this session, a patient coming in with a referral for neck pain. I brought my patient back to a table so we could go through their visit.

"What is your biggest goal that you want to get out of physical therapy?"

"The pain in my neck, I want to get rid of it!" The patient pointed aggressively at their neck, staring intensely at me as they did so.

"Okay, tell me about what things you're not able to do functionally because of your pain?"

My patient paused for effect, stood up from the table, and started rapidly listing off things, aggressively slapping one hand with his fist and continuing to stare intensely at me.

"Sex! Exercise! Work! I can't do my work! I can't do my personal training! I put everything on hold! This shit hurts all the time, man! It's a 10/10, and I **NEED** to get **RID** of it!"

As he was speaking, he walked a lap around the treatment table before aggressively sitting back down, staring intensely at me once more awaiting my response. Clearly, this patient brought a lot of energy with them to the visit, and I felt as if their intense gaze was going straight to my soul. I was not expecting this for my first patient of the day at 8 AM. Then again, I had seen enough people come my way that I partially accepted that just about anything goes in healthcare. I was a little nervous, but at the same time, I made the effort to match his energy as we continued with the rest of the patient interview, the physical exam, and subsequent treatment. For this patient, I was not entirely sure what was contributing to their symptoms primarily and therefore ended up spending too much of the session performing testing rather than choosing a treatment direction as a starting point. In the end, the patient and I seemed to be off to a good start, although I knew that probably would not last if I couldn't figure out what was going on with them.

For this patient's second visit, I was able to focus more on committing to a treatment direction. When we had finished with the visit, I asked the patient, "Do you have any questions for me?" They replied, "I don't have any questions, but I wanted to show you this!"

My patient then proceeded to pull out a pair of nunchucks from their backpack and excitedly hand them to me so that I could hold it. They told me that right after this visit, they were going to go to the local park to practice their combat skills. This was admittedly the first time ever that I encountered someone bringing a melee weapon with them to show me, and I am still not entirely sure how I will react if there is a second time in my career.

~

In a subsequent mentoring session, Kenny and I were reviewing the medical chart for the patient scheduled for my evaluation. The patient was coming to physical therapy for post-surgical management of an ankle fracture that seemed to be improving without any particular complications. From a purely diagnostic standpoint, this should have been a relatively straightforward evaluation. Kenny turned to me and said, "Your goal is to finish the evaluation in 45 minutes." That seemed reasonable enough considering that evaluations had 60 minutes allotted and I already knew what their diagnosis was, therefore saving me the time that would be spent asking diagnostic questions.

I walked to the waiting area and called my patient's name. My patient, who was sitting in a wheelchair, slowly wheeled themselves towards me. This was the first red flag to go off in my head, as this patient's ankle fracture had occurred months before this evaluation and the recent notes from their physician had cleared the patient to begin walking already with full weight bearing about a month prior to this visit. Normally, I would introduce myself in the beginning to the patient. I had zero chance to do so though, as my patient proceeded to babble a non-stop stream of words.

> "You know, I've been working really hard on taking care of my body and I've just been so blessed by my doctor that they've done such a good job taking care of me, and you know I've been taking a lot of vitamins and minerals… Did you know that vitamins and minerals are good for you? You know, I take vitamin D, calcium, collagen… Collagen! You know, people don't believe enough in that stuff, but I'm a really big believer in it, and you know, I'm a really big believer in glucosamine too, I heard it does wonders for your joints and your bones and I'm a really big believer in homeopathy and therapy! You know, I really believe in the miracle of God being able to heal my body with homeopathy…"

My patient continued to ramble non-stop about vitamins, homeopathy, their work as a missionary, the miracles of God and Jesus, and various other random topics not related to their ankle fracture. While I am not opposed in any way, shape, or form to people putting their faith in God and Jesus, I was under some time constraints to obtain information in order to evaluate this person's ankle and get them some good treatment for Day 1.

About 10 minutes into the visit and with zero questions asked by me as of yet, my patient finally asked me, "I don't think I asked you what your name is, what's your name? Derek? Okay that's a good name Derek, I'll pray to God for you. You know, I've been all over the world, I've been to all different parts of Asia, Japan, China, and you know I'm just curious, what kind of Asian are you?"

I was not expecting to be questioned this morning about "what kind of Asian I was." I attempted to redirect the conversation towards asking pertinent questions about their living situation, current level of function, and goals for physical therapy. Most of my attempts were absolutely worthless as the patient was not acknowledging the questions I asked. At one point, I repeated the patient's name multiple times until I got their attention as a form of a hard conversation redirect attempt, before directly saying, "Tell me about (insert whatever important information I needed)." This type of hard conversation redirect worked for 99% of the other patients that I attempted it with. This patient however remained completely unfazed, continuing to ramble endlessly about the benefits of fish oils for Omega 3's, and random memories from their time working as a missionary as they stared off into space.

This patient also knew that I had an observer, Kenny, who was supposed to join us (I informed them ahead of time that we would have an observer). She would peer off to the side to see if she could figure out which clinician standing in our vicinity was Kenny. Off to the side observing and trying his best not to interfere, Kenny could tell that I was not only trying my hardest to obtain clinically useful information, but also that this patient encounter was unfolding as an absolute dumpster fire. The patient kept looking over at Kenny trying to get his attention, and Kenny knew that if he didn't walk over to at least say something briefly, I was going to go nowhere with my patient interview or evaluation.

Kenny walked over to briefly introduce himself, and the patient said, "Oh, your name is Kenny, you know that's a good name too, I'll pray to God for you too for your well-being. You know, I worked as a missionary and traveled all around Asia." My patient looked at me, "I forgot to ask, what kind of Asian are you?" They turned to Kenny, "What kind of Asian are you?" Neither Kenny nor I answered the question, and the patient said, "Oh well, anyways, all Asians are the same," before continuing to ramble more about vitamins and missionary work.

In my clinical practice up to this point, most instances of racism directed towards me were a little more subtle. This took the cake now however and earned the spot of one of the most overt forms of racism directed towards me in a clinical encounter that I've ever experienced.

The patient continued to ramble endlessly about random items unrelated to their ankle fracture as I kept struggling immensely to get the patient to pay attention long enough to follow my directions for examination and treatment. I ended up going 5 minutes over the scheduled 60 minutes. The only physical exam measures that I accomplished were measuring 2 directions of range of motion and treatment consisted of prescribing 2 exercises to do at home that the patient did not do correctly during the session. After the evaluation ended and the patient left, I sat in my chair in disbelief, still trying to process the rollercoaster of an evaluation that had just unfolded.

"Kenny... what in the world just happened?"

"That... That was not your fault... At all. At first, I was writing down some feedback for you to consider during the session with teaching exercises, but, as the session kept going, I was like 'Ohhh noo...' I knew it was especially *not* going well because the patient kept trying to look over at me to get me to come over and was ignoring you. This might be the type of patient where you pick one thing per visit and focus on one thing at a time."

This ended up being really good advice for this patient, and for the duration of my time treating this patient, I would choose one thing at a time to focus on to keep encounters as best organized as I could. I suppose as a positive takeaway, the patient ended up gradually improving with their function throughout my time working with them, and they always expressed gratitude towards me for all of the help that I provided.

March 2021, The Continuation of Trimester 2

Springtime was approaching. The days were gradually getting longer, the workload and challenges of residency continuing to increase in difficulty. At this point in the residency, my cumulative fatigue was mounting. There were a few more memorable patient encounters that stick out in my mind from this month, encounters that occurred over telehealth. Some of them are recounted briefly as follows:

One patient that I evaluated called into their visit from their iPad. As I went through my initial introductions, I noticed that the patient was on public transportation somewhere, most likely on the local train-based rapid transit in the area. On top of us trying to communicate with the patient being on public transit, the patient had a really terrible internet connection, so they kept cutting out every 30 seconds or so. Due to this combination of questionable circumstances, it took me twice as long to perform the patient interview as I normally would have taken. In the process of the patient interview, the patient transitioned from being on the rapid transit, to walking through a transit station, to getting into a taxi, all while continuing to converse with me. Since performing a physical examination of the patient was impossible with my patient sitting in a car, I ended the visit at 30 minutes, requesting them to come in person for their next visit.

BUILDING A LIGHT

I had another patient being evaluated for her shoulder post-surgery. As we went through our exam, we talked about her independence with doing activities of daily living around the house, and how her son was going over to her house to help out with chores around the house due to the surgical precautions for the shoulder. "My son is here helping me with things, but I just want to do them myself! I swear, my son is like Hitler! He's always like, 'Mom, don't do this, mom don't do that! Mom don't use your shoulder!' But I tell you, he's a good boy, He's a very good boy, and I love him. I bet you're a good boy too! You're doing this wonderful job helping people like me!" I will admit, I was not expecting my patient to refer to her son as Hitler-like, nor was I expecting to be called a "good boy." My patient also accidently fell during her evaluation but was able to roll sideways and guard her post-operative shoulder. I asked her if she was okay and she said, "Oh, don't worry about me! I know exactly how to fall! Many years playing soccer, you know how the guys fake their falls in soccer? I've spent many years doing the same thing so don't even sweat it, I know how to protect myself!" This was interspersed with some Spanish that I did not understand but the gist I was getting for this patient's personality was big energy overall.

Two of the most memorable encounters this month both had a common theme: an unexpectedly positive impression of the encounter expressed by the patient. These encounters were reminders that even if I try to predict something with my best judgment, sometimes the results will still surprise me.

For the first encounter, my patient was about to do physical therapy for their first time ever for rehabilitation of their ankle. Prior to the encounter, they had sent a long message to their doctor regarding their expectations for physical therapy. I read the message during my chart review, and there were long explanations regarding how they didn't want to waste time with a video visit, that they would rather come in person, that telehealth as a whole was not worth the initial energy. I had already had a few encounters with previous patients who had expressed similar sentiments, some of whom had screamed at me relentlessly or expressed strong discontent with their care because of the nature of the care being delivered virtually. In my head, I was already starting to prepare for the encounter to not go well. Rather than fully accepting it as a loss though, I decided to use this as an opportunity to really connect with the patient and make them feel like the session was valuable.

I entered the encounter and went through the evaluation with the patient. As we transitioned from the patient interview to the physical exam, I set my laptop up on the ground so that the patient could have a clear view of my ankles to follow along with my tests. "You have the same socks as I do from Costco!" I looked again at my socks, and then at my patient's socks, and we were both wearing identical socks. We proceeded to chat for a minute about the comfiness of the socks, the affordability, and the joy that one can have in their life from good socks. Throughout the evaluation, we also connected on a variety of other non-physical therapy related topics, such as a mutual love for running, mutual love for traveling, and favorite places in the area to get high quality burritos. After discussing exercises and scheduling for the next visit, we had a few minutes left at the end for questions.

> "So, that's all of the items I wanted to check in on with you, for our first visit, what kind of questions do you have about your ankle or physical therapy as a whole?
>
> The patient excitedly said to me, "I don't have any questions right now, but I just want to say that I had such a good experience doing this visit with you! I'm surprised at how well it went, and I felt like it was really convenient!"

I was pleasantly surprised to hear this, and I was happy that I could provide a session that was not only clinically useful but also valuable to the patient. They ended up being very receptive to continuing physical therapy over telehealth and did very well overall with their outcomes and rehabilitation. It was a striking reminder that when I review a patient's medical chart, sometimes I begin to form biases in my head. Implicit bias is often unavoidable, but the conscious effort to keep tabs on it and actively address it can help minimize its impact on the clinical encounter.

For the second encounter, I was evaluating a patient for their chronic low back pain. They had an ongoing history of a rare type of cancer, and much of my initial evaluation with the patient was spent doing medical screening to determine if they would benefit from physical therapy regarding their primary concerns, or if they required medical care outside of physical therapy to be successfully treated. As I proceeded through my patient interview and conversed with the patient, I found it challenging to navigate as some of the answers from the patient were ambiguous, and other answers lined up with information that was concerning enough to me to prompt further questioning. One thing that really stuck out to me from a screening standpoint was that the patient felt like they were having frequent falls, and the week I evaluated them, they reported having fallen 3 times. Their increased frequency in falls started a couple years prior, and they noted that prior to the falls, they would get a feeling of tiredness, vision changes, dizziness, headaches, and lightheadedness. The patient had not personally drawn together the connection between their symptoms and their falls until I highlighted the connection to them. After more discussion, we only had time for a limited physical examination and a little bit of treatment as I spent quite a bit of time discussing the importance of possible referral back to their referring physician for additional evaluation.

"Do you have any other questions or concerns that I can address for you today?"

The patient paused for a moment as they gathered their thoughts. "I'm just overwhelmed…"

Dang it! I talked too much! Or maybe, I think that I talked too much? The patient had a very different follow-up from what I had initially assumed, however.

"I'm just overwhelmed with gratitude. I can really see that you take into consideration a holistic approach with your care. My previous doctors were ones I had for many years, and they weren't really thorough with checking me whenever I went in for annual exams."

The words sunk in, imprinting themselves in my memory as I took the time to truly appreciate their feedback.

Sometimes, the most important thing that a patient needs in the clinical encounter is not a perfect, 100% accurate diagnosis or the textbook best treatment. Sometimes, the most important thing that the patient needs is to believe that their provider cares for them, and that their provider considers them as a whole. The patient needs the secure assurance that their provider considers them as they are, a fellow human being trying to navigate life's uncertainties and challenges. For this patient, the light that they needed for the first day of working together, was a thorough conversation assuring them that their whole self was being thoughtfully considered.

CHAPTER 11

Atlanta

MARCH 2021

Every Wednesday morning during the second trimester, the routine was the same: I would wake up at 6 AM, get ready for the day, and then walk over to the clinic to begin my mentoring session at 7 AM. On Wednesday March 17th, the morning started off just like every other Wednesday morning. I woke up at 6 AM, got ready for the day, and then walked over to the clinic to begin my mentoring session at 7 AM. This morning, I had the chance to watch the sun rise on another Wednesday morning.

A friend of mine texted me to ask me if I was doing okay, that they were reading some news of a shooting in Atlanta the night before. During a gap in patient care, I had a chance to check the news, only to be stunned by the account of eight people dying in a shooting, six of them being Asian.[23] As I read the accounts of the shooting in Atlanta, the feeling of a heavy weight began to form in my chest and stomach. I didn't have enough time to process all of my feelings and thoughts before I had to see my next patient though, so I tried to set it all aside as best as I could to save the processing for later. I soon found out that it was challenging to navigate patient care. My mind would not fully concentrate on the patients in front of me as it would drift off to thinking about the shooting at least once or twice during each patient consult. I knew I wasn't bringing my best clinical care to the clinic that day. I found it hard to do so.

This month, prior to the shooting in Atlanta, I had called my parents recently to let them know how things were going in residency. We talked about residency, general life things, and about my morning runs. Many times, my parents would tell me on our phone calls to be careful on my morning runs. Most of the time, it was to watch for cars. The most recent time, it was different.

> "You have to be careful, especially with the recent violence against Asian people."

I would tell them that I would be okay, that I would make sure to be careful. I would tell them to be careful too of course. Reflecting on that entire Wednesday and especially on the Wednesday morning, I was so incredibly blessed to be able to watch the sunrise on another Wednesday morning. The same could not be said for the eight people in Atlanta who died the night before.

That evening, when I arrived back to my apartment, I couldn't stop thinking about the shooting. I thought about my elderly Chinese American patient in the Fall trimester who had to take the bus to the clinic and did not feel safe riding the bus after dark. I thought about how this shooting was a dark reminder of life outside the clinic and the pursuit of residency.

Questions weighed on my mind. No matter how selfless I was, no matter how much my family and I contributed to society, no matter how hard we worked, would there still be people who placed little to no value on my life because of the way I looked, because of my culture, because of the portrayal in media of people who looked like me? Could people change for the better? Would there always be people that felt enabled by the systemic racism interwoven into the fabric of our country to commit horrendous acts of violence? The rise of hate crimes against Asian Americans throughout 2020 and into 2021 led me to ask the questions of: "What if?" What if it happens to me? To my family? To close friends? To colleagues? To my patients? It hurt my heart to ask these questions and yet, I felt that I could not avoid asking these questions. While I am a believer that people can be innately good and have the capacity to change their hearts for the better, times like this still greatly saddened me and made me wonder.

I had little doubt that many of my patients who emigrated from Asia, or had family of Asian descent, were hurting in their hearts in a similar way that I was. Considering this piece, I kept thinking about how I could best process my thoughts and feelings in a healthy manner that allowed me the space to manage my emotions while trying to still take care of my patients and continuing to be a present support for healing in their lives. It was not easily achieved. It prominently highlighted how caretakers, both professional and personal, carry burdens in their hearts even as they try to care for those around them.

CHAPTER 12

The Second LPE

April 2021

The end of the second trimester was starting to creep up steadily, and with it, the second Live Patient Examination. This time, I knew more of what to expect with regards to the entire flow of the LPE. The knowledge did not put me at ease however, and I was instead starting to stress over the LPE. The standard to pass this time was much higher at 80%, and I couldn't help but think about how much I had struggled on my first LPE. A part of me feared having another patient who was equally ambiguous in responding to my questions as the patient had been during my first LPE. The stress led me to doing more preparation ahead of time with not only reviewing the medical chart for my patient, but also building an entire spreadsheet of information. I included all the possible pertinent anatomical structures that could be involved, associated questions, physical exam tests and all other information that I could think of. For the second LPE, my proctors were Kenny and the residency coordinator Cathy, who was also my upcoming mentor for Trimester 3 of residency.

My patient came to the clinic with a referral for evaluation of their ankle. The timing of this patient with their referral was interesting because later in the same week, we had a course on advanced management of the foot and ankle scheduled.

As the examination began, I asked the patient to map out what places they had their symptoms. They pointed to three different distinct parts of their foot and ankle. As I continued to proceed through the examination, I noted differences in their answers.

At the end of the patient interview, I stepped aside with the proctors. I felt like I had a better-quality diagnosis list this time around.

"So, what is your current ranking for your hypotheses?"

"Well, their symptoms and overall history are most consistent with a chronic lateral ankle ligament sprain, my secondary hypothesis is Achilles tendinopathy, and my third hypothesis is plantar fasciopathy."

I also provided my standing rationale based on the information provided by the patient for each hypothesis that I considered. I felt nervous, but my list felt semi-reasonable to me as I had one item to cover each of the three specific areas that the patient pointed to for their pain. As I proceeded through the physical examination, my internal feelings of anxiety continued to build. Still, I at least had seemingly more tangible hypotheses that I could objectively assess and thought that I had somewhat covered my bases during the physical examination. After the physical examination, the proctors asked me again about any changes to my thought process.

"So, any changes to your hypothesis list?" With provision of rationale from the physical examination and patient history combined, I provided my new list. I still had chronic lateral ankle ligament sprain as my first choice, but my secondary and tertiary hypotheses had swapped places.

THE SECOND LPE

"Okay, do you know which ligament of the ankle for the ankle sprain?"

My mind froze for what seemed like a minute. Did I even check the ligaments properly? How do I even check ankle ligaments? It was a reminder that under extensive stress, the mind tended to not recall otherwise foundational information. It was not until later in the week after the LPE that I reviewed how to assess the major ligaments on the outside of the ankle and realized that I had forgotten to add in specific stress testing for the ankles. Doing stress testing on the ankle to better isolate the ligaments would have taken no more than a minute, yet that would have provided me some useful information for improving the precision of my diagnosis and potentially better individualizing the treatment plan for this patient.

I conceded to Kenny and Cathy that I couldn't remember. A weight formed in my chest again as I proceeded through treatment, trying to find something that would be meaningful to the patient as well as objectively helpful for the patient. Due to a combination of poor in-the-moment reasoning and stress, I ended up choosing treatment to address one of my alternate diagnoses rather than directly addressing my main hypothesis.

After the documentation time frame, I proceeded through the oral defense with Cathy and Kenny. As a whole, my rationale on the oral defense had improved in quality compared to my first live patient examination. However, after reflecting on feedback from both proctors, I realized just how inadequate the actual evaluation portion had been, and acknowledged that the examination was subpar compared to other examinations I had performed previously. I still felt as a whole during this stage of residency that my diagnostic abilities and rationale for consistently choosing the best treatment to address my hypothesis was still not quite where I wanted it to be. I didn't learn until during the feedback portion of the LPE that

I should have either focused on one primary symptom area and made the diagnosis list for that one area, or I should have developed 3 different lists of diagnoses for the 3 different areas of pain that the patient reported. As a resident at this stage, I had nowhere near the mental capacity to build 3 different diagnostic lists, but it was something of perceived value to consider for the future.

At the end of the oral defense, I asked my proctors what would happen next, whether this was a passing result or if I would need to retake the LPE.

> "Well, we have to count up your points and discuss a little further about the scoring for your examination this time around. It's clear that you've improved since your first LPE, but there are some things that we would expect more of by this stage of the residency."

A day or so after the LPE, Cathy requested to meet virtually with myself and Kenny. After further discussion between the two of them, they concluded that my performance on the LPE was insufficient to pass, and that I would have to retake the LPE in a month's time. Both of them could tell that I was disappointed but accepting of the result and encouraged me to view the retake as another opportunity to highlight my clinical skills. Kenny added an additional note during our virtual meeting:

> "A lot of this second trimester was really working on patient rapport and connecting with your patients. While this will be helpful for your career as a physical therapist, it does not necessarily directly improve the diagnostic capabilities that residency tends to look for. You have demonstrated growth since the beginning of the trimester, and we know that you have the capacity based on your progression in the last few

THE SECOND LPE

months and from what I've observed during our mentoring sessions."

I thanked both Cathy and Kenny for taking time out of their schedules to meet again. The meeting ended shortly thereafter with all of us logging off of Zoom. I closed my laptop, thoughts racing through my head as I processed my overall well-being, the gravity of the conversation, and my cumulative fatigue. I was now in a position where I not only had to attend to all of my original designated residency responsibilities, but I now had an extra LPE to add on. I had also started residency with a long-term low back injury that had been gradually building in its pain intensity, impacting both my physical function and mental ability to focus.

As a whole, the failure of the second LPE at the end of the second trimester was a tough result to accept. Although I had grown in the last few months in my ability to connect with patients and make them feel cared for, there were still plenty of shortcomings I faced. I did not feel as if I had time to feel sorry for myself, however. There were still responsibilities to attend to with residency and patients to treat. Life continued to move forward, impartial to my personal struggles and successes.

PART 3

The Third Trimester

Typically, the transition to the third trimester of residency is marked by both the completion of the second LPE and the transition towards the third mentor. In my case, I was transitioning to my third mentor, Cathy. However, because I did not pass the second LPE, I would have to retake it. While from a calendar timeline standpoint I was in the third trimester, mentally it did not feel like I was in the third trimester. In my mind, I had to pass the retake of the second LPE before I could say that I was in the third trimester.

Based on the framework laid out by Harvey in the Fall, the theme of this trimester of residency was supposed to be the "building back up" of the resident; the trimester where everything comes together. For me, an additional theme of this trimester was putting together my ability to not only build a strong hypothesis list for anatomical sources of someone's symptoms, but to also begin to be able to build a parallel ranking list for prioritizing the most important items to treat to address my primary hypothesis. As a resident, orchestrating the simultaneous ranking of hypotheses and treatment items in real-time demanded nothing short of dialed-in mental gymnastics. In this regard, Cathy served a critical role in guiding me with organizing my thought process throughout these final few months.

Within my residency experience, each trimester felt more challenging than the last. This trimester would be, by far, the most challenging one. My cumulative fatigue had been steadily building through the calendar year, but exponentially increased during this trimester. My long-term low back injury was also progressively worsening through residency, adding another layer of challenge to the trimester. Through the next few months, there would be a lot of self-doubt, stress, anxiety, and questions about self-worth. Not passing my second LPE imposed an extra source of stress that weighed on my mind. In retrospect, it is no surprise that my physical symptoms started to worsen in parallel with the compounding fatigue and stress. If I were to give physical therapy residents in similar circumstances a single piece of advice, it would be this: your self-worth and positive impact on patients' lives is not defined by your failures or struggles. The greatest challenges of residency had yet to come.

CHAPTER 13

The Second LPE Round 2

May 2021

It had been eight months since residency began in September, 2020, and 14 months since COVID-19 was declared a public emergency in March of the same year. Outside of the turmoil of residency, things were changing with the pandemic. Deaths and cases were trending downward in the US but surging upward in India.[24,25] At the local level, restaurants and businesses were gradually opening up more than they had earlier in the year.[26] As the days lengthened and the sun shined longer, life seemed a little brighter.

In the grand scheme of life, four months is but a fraction of time that a person spends living life. The contextual factors in a person's life however can profoundly impact their perception of the passage of time. As I entered the third trimester and looked ahead, the four months remaining seemed so little time yet so daunting. It felt like I had a lifetime of work stretched out in front of me, and I thought that maybe somehow, it would all be compacted together with the resulting knowledge learned along the way taken to heart. There were still many major challenges to overcome, both known and unanticipated. The first one of course was the retake of the second LPE.

BUILDING A LIGHT

The retake was scheduled later in the month, which meant that I had a chance to go through some mentoring with Cathy. Over the course of the month, Cathy now took over Kenny's role of observing me treat patients, recording feedback, and discussing patient cases with me.

On the day of the LPE retake, I felt an extra heightened level of nerves. On one hand, I had another month's worth of patient care and mentoring under my belt to bring to the table. On the other hand, this was a retake and if I failed this retake, I would go on probation and likely be in a precarious situation for continuing residency. I tried not to think about the implications of failing, focusing instead on the types of questions I would ask and possible diagnoses for consideration based on the patient's medical chart. Was I ready? Did my proctors think I was ready?

Kenny walked into the back office where I was doing last minute preparations, and with a smile said, "You ready to kick ass?" Clearly, Kenny was not too worried about me, and that put me a little more at ease (as a side note, spending the pandemic with everyone wearing masks, I learned that you could tell when someone's smiling by the way their eyes move).

We walked out into the clinic space to a designated area for the LPE retake. As I was sitting with Kenny and Cathy waiting for my patient, both of them checked in to see how I was feeling.

"How are you feeling?"

"A little nervous, but about as ready as I'll be."

"Trust your knowledge of the anatomy. We've seen you do evaluations before, and we know that you can logically organize information presented. We're not concerned for you, we know that you're there."

THE SECOND LPE ROUND 2

This was a reassuring last reminder before I began the LPE. I was still feeling a little nervous, but I kept telling myself to trust my knowledge, to trust in the process I had been working on for all these concentrated months — with the extra challenges of clinical work in a hospital system during a global pandemic. Sometimes, all you can do in a situation with a lot of variables is to focus on the variables that you can control.

The LPE retake began shortly thereafter. I started my patient on time, a person who had been referred for back pain with accompanying nerve related symptoms. As I proceeded through my patient interview, I found the patient to be wordier with their answers to my questions than I anticipated. Because of this, I ended up taking about 25 minutes on the patient interview. After the patient interview, I stepped aside with Kenny and Cathy to provide my top hypotheses for anatomical contributors for this patient's pain. We also discussed how much the symptoms were affecting the patient, the degree to which the symptoms could be reproduced and calmed down, the timeline of the injury and whether it was improving, staying the same or getting worse. I had initially rated this patient's symptoms as being on the milder end for their symptom irritability, which on paper meant that I could proceed with a more aggressive physical exam.

We returned to the patient, and I started my physical exam. I started with having the patient walk and squat. As the patient was moving, I started to realize that maybe I was wrong in my initial assessment and that the intensity of their pain was much higher than I had initially thought. I transitioned over to assessing their range of motion.

"Okay, let's have you bend forward as if you're trying to touch your toes."

"HNHGNHNUHN" The patient grimaced and groaned as they tried to bend forward. Internally, I cringed as I watched the patient. I could tell that this was super painful for them to do.

"Uh, okay, let's have you come back up, and lean back as far as you can comfortably."

"HNJNGNNGN" The patient grimaced and groaned some more as they tried to lean back. This was also clearly super painful for them to do.

The rest of the testing for their active range of motion was also really painful. By now, it was clear to me that they were in a lot of pain with just simple movement, and I had severely underestimated their symptom irritability. Mentally, I was starting to cut down on tests, to save them for their next visit, trying my best to prioritize the things that I would check for this first day.

I moved the patient to the table to have them lie on their back. As I attempted to perform a lower extremity neurological screen of their sensation, muscle function and reflexes, I could tell that it was very difficult to get a clean assessment of their muscle function given how irritable their symptoms were. Despite this challenge, I was still able to gather some important information related to the testing for my hypotheses. One other useful piece of information that I picked up on during the testing was that when this patient brought their knee towards their chest, this improved their pain. I made a mental note to come back to this information in a little bit.

I proceeded through the rest of my physical examination, checking the joint mobility of the low back before repositioning the patient on their back with their knees bent for comfort. I checked with my patient to make sure that they were comfortable before

THE SECOND LPE ROUND 2

stepping aside again with Cathy and Kenny to discuss any changes to my hypotheses.

At this point, I had enough information to make some changes to my hypothesis list and gave them my rankings. With regard to my top choice, Kenny asked me, "Any conflicting information that you gathered during your exam?"

I carefully thought for a moment about my top choice and any information in the exam that contradicted it. The image of the patient bringing their knee to their chest to stretch popped back up in my head. "Well, the patient said that when they position themselves in hip flexion, that position improves their symptoms, which would not necessarily line up with my primary choice."

Shortly after, Kenny, Cathy and I walked back over to my patient. I had just 15 minutes to go in the allotted 60 minutes. I had to make my time and treatment count. Thinking more about what my patient had told me, I decided to commit to trying exercises that would have them intentionally round out their low back. I chose two exercises, checking their range of motion and pain levels after teaching each exercise. After the patient improved in both pain and range of motion with the first exercise, I knew that I was on-track for treating this patient successfully on day 1. As a bonus, the patient also responded well to the second exercise that I provided.

At the end of the evaluation and documentation period, I went through the oral defense with Cathy and Kenny. I felt like my physical exam was nowhere near as efficient as it could have been. However, I was able to discuss which items I chose to prioritize and offer a logical rationale for my choices during the evaluation and treatment. After the formal oral defense portion, we transitioned into more feedback related to the case.

Kenny: "One thing that we were really happy to see this time around was that we could tell you were actively reflecting throughout the process and trying to actively problem solve as you went through the exam."

Cathy: "Yeah, definitely agree on that, we could see that there was more reflection in action during this exam compared to your other LPE, and it's more in line with what we would expect for residents at this stage of the year."

Both of them acknowledged that this was a pretty tough case due to the patient's heightened symptom intensity, which made it difficult to gather clean information. Additionally, conflicting pieces of information presented in the patient's narrative and attained in the physical exam contributed to the lack of a clean primary diagnosis that I could commit to. Despite these challenges though, I was still able to navigate through the evaluation and provide meaningful treatment that was able to help the patient on Day 1. After full discussion and feedback, it was the moment of truth. Did I pass the exam? Or did I fail again?

"So, as of right now, you either passed, or barely passed." Kenny smiled at me as he said this. "Worst case scenario is, you barely passed."

Cathy added to it: "What Kenny's saying is that we still have to add up the scores of course, but you most likely passed."

I let out a sigh of relief. It was reassuring to know that I was still on track with what was expected out of residents by this stage of the residency. It was also a humbling reminder that I still had such a long way to go with growing as a clinician. Kenny and Cathy totaled the points, and it turned out that I had passed with a score of at least 80%. Despite this win, I still felt a sense of being on edge as we had more major examinations coming up in June. There was just a brief moment of time for me to come up for air, take a deep breath, and descend back into the tumultuous depths of residency, where nothing can be taken for granted and professional composure and exam performances are ever susceptible to residency's capricious currents. Nevertheless, in a moment of achievement, I had passed LPE 2 the second time around. There were still many more challenges to come.

CHAPTER 14

The Second Technique Practical Exam and Written Exam

June 2021

Summer had arrived. Dense fog permeated the city of San Francisco, which was fitting to match the mood of this stage of residency. There were now only 3 months to go before the end of residency. The last of our advanced residency courses had concluded, and we were set to be tested on both hands-on treatment and assessment techniques, as well as take a written examination covering all of the course material we had learned since January 2021.

By this point in the residency, I was experiencing multiple symptoms consistent with burnout. Headaches were occurring on a daily basis. Multiple nights in the week, I was having trouble going to sleep, a rare occurrence in my usual daily life. There was never enough sleep or rest. Each day, it was getting a little bit harder to get out of bed, partially due to my exhaustion and partially because lying on my back was the only time my low back did not hurt. Pain from my low back injury was also amplified by the stress, and all of my efforts to self-treat had had limited success. I felt like I was dragging a heavy weight with me to the clinic each day, and the

THE SECOND TECHNIQUE PRACTICAL EXAM AND WRITTEN EXAM

weight would build throughout the day both physically and mentally. Suffice it to say, there was quite a bit of anxiety associated with the overall state of my physical and mental health.

The technique practical examination was first. It was the same format as the first practical, except that the proctors this time were Cathy and Alison. Mariano and I had practiced extensively, staying for hours on end each week after patient care, to ingrain the muscle memory so that we felt at least somewhat ready.

Alison named the first technique, a treatment technique for the ankle, and my mind went blank. Was this it? Why was I spacing out on the technique? Was I really going to fail this because I couldn't get my brain to work on the first of multiple techniques? I had to at least try. I knew we had definitely discussed this particular technique, but the information was not quite coming back to me immediately. *First trimester Derek probably would have given up. Third trimester Derek refused to take another major failure without trying.* I began to set up the technique on Cathy who was serving as the standardized patient. My first time setting up the technique was highly questionable, and I could tell it was highly questionable. Bits and pieces started to come back to my mind however, and I told myself to stay calm as I slowly and methodically worked through the bits and pieces to put the technique together. This same trend occurred for the other techniques being tested: I would partially forget the technique, commit to a partial set-up, and then gradually problem solve in real-time to work towards what I thought was the best possible set-up for the technique being tested. After the end of the technique practical exam, both Cathy and Alison asked me what my thoughts were about how I performed.

"Honestly, I'm not sure if I passed. If I didn't pass, I'm accepting of the need to re-take it. I felt like there was a lot of in-the-moment problem solving that I had to do to set up the techniques."

Alison gave her thoughts on my overall performance: "So, you actually passed the practical, and Cathy and I agreed that what put you over into a passing score was that we could both tell that you were able to reflect in the moment to actively problem solve, and that's what we're looking for in the residents by this stage of the year. We were a *little* concerned when you were setting up the first technique, but we could see you gradually piece things together and put together something pretty close to the proper set-up."

I had put the technique practical examination successfully behind me but did not feel at all relieved. I had just performed some of my best real-time problem solving of residency thus far just to barely push through with each technique name not ringing any bells as I began my exam. Burnout is a very unforgiving companion in residency, one that exacts a steady toll on a person's memory and ability to perform at their highest level. Our written exam was coming up, and I felt very inadequately prepared for it.

On the day of the written examination, I logged onto Zoom to meet with Mariano and Alison to complete the examination. As I worked my way through the exam, many of the questions seemed more multi-layered or precise beyond what I had studied, and I felt a sense of uncertainty cloud my mind throughout the exam. After Mariano and I completed the examination, we had a couple of days to wait until the results came out. The passing score of the written exam was 80%. I had only scored less than 75%. Because of this, I would have to retake the examination.

Admittedly, I was disappointed that I had failed the written exam. There was still the opportunity to retake the exam of course,

THE SECOND TECHNIQUE PRACTICAL EXAM AND WRITTEN EXAM

but that would not happen until after our scheduled week-long break at the end of the month. This was now my second major failure of residency. When our break arrived, I traveled back to my home for the week and elected to stay home for the entire week, pouring all of my time into studying. Over the course of the week, I poured dozens of hours into studying the material from courses in depth, trying to cover it all as best as I could. I had already reached close to total burnout and found myself trying to search the depths of my mind for something, anything that would help me retain information. My headspace was becoming clouded, a dense fog of stress spreading throughout and taking hold in lieu of useful clinical information.

I committed almost all of my remaining motivation, grit, and memory into studying, hoping that it would be enough to pass the retake of the examination.

CHAPTER 15

Digging Through Fog

July 2021

When one fully commits themselves physically, mentally, and emotionally to a particular endeavor, it is a gamble. When it feels like it works out, it can be incredibly rewarding. When it feels like the efforts are for nothing, it can be incredibly crushing. Typically, by this stage of the residency, most of the exams and testing are behind the residents and the work is supposed to become more manageable. This trimester thus far was not the lighter load that I needed from a personal health perspective. Instead, it felt as if the work was continuing to relentlessly crush me, the cumulative fatigue of the last few months slowly dragging me down.

After a completely mentally draining week-long hiatus, I returned to residency for the retake of the written exam. The written exam had fewer questions, but the passing score was still 80% so the margin of error was smaller. I proceeded through the exam intentionally, answering the questions as best as I could and hoping that my additional studying would pay off.

Shortly after taking the exam, I found out the results through an email from Alison. I opened my computer and email and read through the email.

I didn't pass the retake of the written exam. My score was 78%. I had missed passing by one point. That point could have been found anywhere and nowhere on the exam day.

This was now my third major failure of residency, and I was now on academic probation. The weight of my current status gnawed at my sense of self-worth.

Later in the same week, I met with Alison to discuss a remediation plan. Alison shared the proposal with me, which included five different components to it. In order to complete it, I had to do the following:

– Self-correction with clinical rationale for the exam questions that I had missed.

– Review of a monograph on a weekly basis for orthopedic care of different regions of the body up until the week of taking a practice orthopedic clinical specialty exam planned for August.

– Create residency level test questions based on the monographs.

– Score above a certain designated threshold for a practice orthopedic clinical specialty exam.

– Pass the final LPE (which I had to do regardless to finish residency in general).

As she explained the proposal, I felt an internal conflict within myself grow. On one side of the internal conflict, there were intrusive thoughts entering my mind that the amount of work in contrast to the one-point margin by which I did not pass the exam retake was very disproportionate. To a part of me, this multi-part plan represented more work for my already burnt-out self to attend to, more weight to pull down the sinking ship that represented my overall health in multiple dimensions.

On the other side of the internal conflict was reflection on the long-term reasoning for this plan. As I read through the proposal and asked questions for clarification, I also used that time to try to set aside my negative thoughts about the proposal. The ultimate goal of residency was not to just pass exams, go through the motions and complete the residency. One of the goals was to be ready to pass the clinical specialty exam that I would take next year, but the more important goal was to be able to take this information to improve my capacity to treat patients effectively and with dignity in my daily consultations with them. Still, the remediation proposal seemed daunting. In the end, the side of me reflecting on the long-term benefit of the proposal won out, and we agreed on the proposal.

Through much of the month of July, I felt like I was slowly drowning, sinking under the standard expected of the residency. The quality of my patient care as a whole was suffering greatly. Personal life events and worsening low back pain were also contributing to my overall stress, and the cumulative burnout severely affected my ability to function in the clinic. Often, it was hard to remember information. My headspace felt fuzzy, my mind foggy. There were many times during visits when I would ask my patient a question and would promptly forget what question I had asked. There were other times I would ask my patient a question and would remember the question, but when the patient would give their answer, the response would only register in my mind as sound coming out of their mouth rather than a coherent answer, forcing me to ask the question again to understand their response. Sometimes, I would forget how to do some basic examination measures. Other times, I would forget what treatment I was going to provide.

My relatively upbeat first few months of residency now felt like little more than a distant dream from a different lifetime.

I had multiple patients during this time with highly complex backgrounds and I was struggling immensely to treat them successfully. Despite my best efforts, many of these patients did not improve in their conditions and they left, disappointed in me. The consecutive stream of failure to help these patients disheartened me greatly. I felt like my work didn't matter, that my efforts were worthlessly expended in a bottomless pit. I felt trapped within myself. I felt like I had been constantly playing catch-up since April. I felt like I was trying my very best, and yet my best just wasn't good enough. Not enough for my patients. Not enough for myself. Certainly not enough for the program it seemed. I started to wonder if this was it, if I was going to fail out of residency because I was just not enough. I simultaneously wondered if I was even cut out to be a physical therapist. Completion of the residency seemed to be slowly drifting out of reach.

There were weeks on end when even motivating myself to get out of bed was difficult because of how discouraged I felt. Massive headaches were a daily occurrence. I took too long to fall asleep and would have to wake up too soon. Some days, I didn't know whether I wanted to scream or cry. Other days I just wanted to crawl into my bed and do nothing else but sleep to avoid all of my responsibilities. It was hard to think about the next day, the next week, the next patient.

Towards the end of July, Mariano and I presented case reports of patients and topics we had been working on since the beginning of residency. Typically, the presentation of the case report for the residents was supposed to mark a point of celebration and excitement, the last big checkpoint before the final LPE. I couldn't find the energy in me to be genuinely excited for the presentation day though. Instead, when I searched within myself, I found only a sense of apathy and exhaustion to bring to the case report presentations layered over by feigned enthusiasm to hide my true feelings from the audience. I didn't feel proud of my presentation. I didn't feel proud of my work. I didn't feel proud to be a resident. I didn't feel proud of myself. The case report was just another thing to do, another task to complete.

The next week after the case report presentations, I was in a mentoring session with Cathy, and we talked briefly about how things in residency were going.

> "How are things going? Do you feel excited to be done with your case report?"

> I shrugged, feeling indifferent to the case report. "Honestly… not really. I know that sounds bad… but it just felt like another thing to be done with. I just… I just feel tired I guess…"

Cathy could tell that the last few weeks burdened me heavily. "Well, even if it is hard to feel like you accomplished something big, it is still a really big achievement to be proud of, and hopefully you'll be able to eventually celebrate it at some point."

It was hard for me at the time to be proud of that case report. I still felt like there was so much to overcome, so much still to complete. All I could think about was getting through one day at a time, putting one foot in front of the other. The *light* I had been trying to build through the year seemed dim, a windblown flutter of flame threatening to be blown out in a vast darkness. I struggled to remember why I started residency, why I had embarked on this journey to begin with.

CHAPTER 16

Remembering Why I Started

In countless conversations with friends and family, whenever I share that I work in healthcare, everyone talks about how wonderful it is that I am in a position to help other people. Oftentimes, patients go to healthcare providers in order to seek help in some form. There are times however, that while the healthcare provider is helping a patient, the patient in turn also helps the provider in a different way. Patients can help healthcare providers rediscover their purpose and passion for their work, time and time again. They can remind healthcare providers of why they entered the healthcare field in the first place. In my journey, I was reminded of why I chose to pursue residency and why I chose this profession.

July – August 2021

I was now 11 months into my year-long residency, an arduous journey made even more challenging, due to being on the frontlines of providing care in a global pandemic: COVID-19. Around the same time frame as the case report presentation, I had a final visit with a patient whom I had been working with for a few months now. We had never met in person, doing all of our physical therapy visits virtually through telehealth. Despite this, we had formed a good working dynamic, and with each visit the patient was gradually improving. At the end of their visit, I asked the patient if they had any last questions or thoughts.

> "Well, I just want to say thank you so much for all of your help. I can say that this is the best I've ever felt about myself in the last 6 years."

A couple days after that final visit I received a message in my medical chart's message inbox:

> "Dear Derek,
> Thank you for treating my pain. Your practitioner skills were well demonstrated as you were very patient in listening to the various symptoms I was experiencing, answering my questions, and providing the correct treatments. Your ability to diagnose and assign treatment has been very successful. I am no longer dependent upon a walking cane, I can walk a mile at an easy pace, and even my headaches have lessened. I am pleased that I can now stand and iron, vacuum my home, and drive my vehicle with no fear or discomfort. Again, thank you for your medical expertise and I'm very grateful to you."

Oftentimes, patients would only use this messaging system for its intended function: to ask questions or provide updates on their care. Never did I anticipate that a patient would use the messaging system to express gratitude for my work, and for that I was grateful. It was one of the notable reminders during this challenging period that my patients were in fact getting better, even if results sometimes took longer than I thought they would take.

REMEMBERING WHY I STARTED

There was one other patient in particular who helped me to reflect once more on the residency journey, a patient I first encountered during a mentoring session. The session started off like all of my other mentoring sessions this trimester: Cathy and I were sitting in the clinic reviewing the medical charts for my patients, discussing my plans, possible hypotheses to consider for the evaluation, and possible treatments based on the hypotheses. For the patient I was going to be evaluating this day, their referral was for long term chronic low back pain.

My patient arrived, and I brought them over to our designated treatment table. We sat down, and the patient began to talk as I attentively listened. As part of our conversation, we got to talking about their level of function and living situation.

> "Tell me about your daily routine. What does that look like for you currently for things that you're doing around the house?"

> "Well, I live alone, so I do all of the chores around the house myself, but my children who live close by can come to help out. I've always been on the go, and I've always wanted to be able to do everything myself."

The patient paused for a moment. Tears began to flow from my patient's eyes. I leaned in a little closer, sensing that this was challenging for the patient to talk about, and it was especially important for me to be present in the moment for this patient.

> "You know, I've been independent my entire life, and I'm just not ready to give that up. My pain makes it hard for me to keep things going though."

BUILDING A LIGHT

More tears flowed from my patient's eyes. I grabbed tissues and handed them to my patient. They thanked me as they wiped their eyes. We talked more about what was important to them and what they wanted to get out of coming to physical therapy.

For the physical exam portion, I had taken longer than I anticipated on the patient interview and therefore ended up cutting out some exam measures to save for the next visit so that I could more rapidly transition towards meaningful treatment for the first day. After treatment, our visit was reaching its end.

"Do you have any questions or any other last things that you would like to share?"

"I just want to say thank you so much for being patient with me, and I'm so sorry I teared up during our session."

"Oh, there's no need to apologize for tears! It is very much okay, and I know that this is something that has been very challenging for you to live with."

The patient departed, and then Cathy and I debriefed the session.

"So, what did you think?"

"Well, I definitely was not as efficient as I wanted to be with the physical examination, so I saved the testing for my alternate diagnoses for day 2. I probably could have done a couple other things in the session differently too, but I think the treatment I provided to address my primary diagnosis was appropriate and helped address the patient's concern. I felt like in my mind I was going back and forth on how much testing to do versus how much time to spend connecting with the patient and went more of the route of trying to connect with the patient today."

Cathy nodded. "I think it's fine for today that you did not get to all the things you could have tested for the physical exam. It was important that you could read that this patient was getting emotional talking about their quality of life, and you took the time to connect with them while still addressing your primary hypothesis. You can always just do the exam measures you didn't cover today at the next visit just to be sure, and then go from there."

Over the course of a few more visits, this patient and I continued to work together, and the patient gradually improved in their function. Unfortunately, this patient's rate of improvement with their pain was not quite what the patient had hoped for despite my best efforts. On the patient's final visit, they shared news with me that they were going to try other treatments instead to address their pain. Rather than being disappointed in me though, they were very grateful as they felt more empowered to do their daily activities despite having pain. They thanked me for my help and had brought me something.

> "I brought you this gift as well as a card!" To my surprise, the patient had thoughtfully brought me a parting gift for me to take home. "I would give you a hug too, but we're still in a pandemic, so an air hug with much love for now will do!"

I thanked the patient for their gift and shortly after, the patient left the clinic. I did not open the card until the end of the workday. As I sat in the back office finishing up my documentation, I decided to take a moment to open the card. I sat back in the chair and read the card.

"Dear Derek,
May your dreams unfold as your strength, your patience and your passion lead you to your next step in your future! Thank you for helping me!"

I read it and reread it, wiping a few tears from my eyes as I stared at the card. It was such a small gesture, yet the genuine heart behind it had such a profound effect on me and touched me deeply. I started to think more about this patient and my other patient who messaged me online. Little did these patients realize the full extent to which their thanks were received. I very much needed their expressions of gratitude at this point in my journey.

There were many times throughout the last few months where my most prominent thoughts fixated on my weaknesses. The times that I fell short. The times that I didn't feel like I was enough. These patients reminded me that even though I was still a "work in progress," I still had the capacity to positively impact their lives and the lives of many other patients in the past, present and future.

I may have brought these patients a *light* to give them hope for navigating their pain, but in turn these patients brought me a *light* to give me a little more courage to keep going.

They were a reminder of why I chose to set out on this residency journey at the outset: To commit to becoming the best clinician and mentor I was capable of becoming. To bring my patients a *light* for navigating their uncertain injuries.

They were a reminder that my work with patients mattered.

They were a reminder that I mattered.

CHAPTER 17

The Final Live Patient Examination

August 2021

The final month of residency had arrived. I had been steadily grinding through the remediation plan over the course of the previous few weeks without any complications. One notable benefit of reviewing the monographs weekly was that I was starting to have some treatment breakthroughs with treating some of my patients using the information that I had reviewed. It was a reminder in real time of the true benefit of going through the remediation plan: gaining the knowledge to treat my patients more effectively. As for the practice clinical specialty exam, I not only passed the score threshold set by Alison but scored one of the highest percentages in the history of the residency. Pieces were starting to come together, no sooner, no later, but right on time. Almost all of the portions of the remediation plan were completed by the middle of the month.

There was one more challenge to overcome of course: The third and final Live Patient Examination. This one was for all the marbles. If I passed, I was set to complete residency on time. If I failed, I would have to extend residency. With the state of my deteriorating physical and mental health by this month, the thought of extending residency would trigger an internal sense of anxiety. I tried as best as I could to set aside that anxiety, focusing on the preparation aspects that were within my control.

For my LPE, my proctors were Cathy and another one of the faculty members, Dean. From the chart review, I was surprised at the amount of information present on the patient's background relative to the previous patients for my other LPEs. My patient was being referred to physical therapy for their knee, and they had a full detailed history regarding their knee pain. Based on the information present in the chart, I found I was able to effectively preplan the questions I wanted to ask, choose possible hypotheses for consideration, and choose possible treatment options to match my hypotheses. Still, there was always room for something unexpected to happen as was the case for every other LPE I had completed.

Test day arrived, and I went to the clinic feeling an elevated level of nerves. As I waited in the back of the clinic with the proctors, both proctors asked me how I was feeling. I admitted that I was a little nervous, but also about as ready as I was going to be.

Cathy: "Just remember the things we've been talking about in mentoring. We know that you're ready, just keep those things in mind as you go through the exam."

Dean leaned forward. "Here, let me fix this for you," and he proceeded to adjust the collar of my button-up shirt to make it more presentable. In my heightened level of nervousness going into this LPE, I had forgotten to adjust my shirt properly. It was probably evident to both Cathy and Dean that I was more than a little nervous going in.

The patient's visit time arrived, and the patient checked in right on time. It was Go Time. I brought the patient back to the testing corner, introduced them to everyone, and then went into my examination flow.

THE FINAL LIVE PATIENT EXAMINATION

"Before we get into our visit here today, what is the most important thing that you would like to get out of physical therapy?"

The patient seemed unsure. "Uh… I want to get rid of my knee pain, I guess. I don't really know otherwise."

"Okay, well, that is something we can definitely work on. We'll talk more about your knee's history, we'll do a physical exam to take a look to see how you're moving, and then we can talk about some exercises for you to do at home to help with your knee."

The patient still seemed unsure. "Oh okay… I don't really know what to expect from physical therapy, and actually I did not think that we were going to do a physical exam today."

As we proceeded through the patient interview, the overall interaction felt a little bit awkward. The answers they gave though were all direct and useful for the most part with giving me the information to capture their full profile. By the end of the patient interview, I had narrowed down my hypothesis list and had planned out the physical exam measures that I wanted to assess.

In residency, one point that was reinforced and something I was constantly working on was being intentional about asking patients to expose skin around the areas where they reported symptoms. This was to get into the habit of refining our observation skills and helping us to pick up on potentially important information that would help us with determining proper treatment.

For this patient, my original plan was to have them change into shorts. The first part that threw me off a little bit was at the end of the patient interview.

"Are you okay with changing into shorts for today's visit? This will help me with being able to thoroughly assess your knee."

"Uhh… No… I think I'm okay… I would like to stay with my regular pants."

That was understandable, but I still needed to have proper visualization of their knee if possible.

"Okay, well are you comfortable with rolling up your pant legs?

"Well, actually, I have two pairs of long pants on, so it's very hard for me to roll up my pants."

As they said this, they rolled up their first pair of long pants to reveal their second pair of long pants. By this point, exposing the knee for proper visual assessment was most likely out of the question. I believed this was the first time anyone had ever come to an evaluation with me wearing multiple pairs of long pants. I tried to see if it was possible to at least get a proper movement assessment of their ankles to see if there were any factors with their ankles contributing to their knee pain.

"Okay, well are you comfortable with taking off your shoes and socks?"

"Uh… I'm not comfortable with taking off my shoes and socks. I don't want to step on the floor."

Guess I was going to have to enter the physical exam and hope that I could pick up all the information I needed without full visualization of the ankles and the knees. I stepped into a side room to discuss my hypotheses with Cathy and Dean, and then stepped back out to proceed through the physical examination.

As I proceeded through my physical examination, I found myself trying very hard to reflect intentionally in the moment, more so than I ever had during previous LPEs. As I reflected, I made appropriate adjustments for my examination and treatment. For this patient, I was able to observe multiple key items likely contributing to their knee pain, perform pertinent testing to cover my hypotheses, and choose seemingly appropriate exercises to provide for their first day. There was only one part that threw off my train of thought again during the physical exam, which occurred during my strength testing for assessing their hip and thigh muscle strength. During this portion, when I asked the patient to transition from lying on their side to lying on their stomach, they could not figure out my directions on how I wanted them to be positioned. It took me what felt like a minute or two to get the patient to lie on their stomach as they proceeded to lie on their side, then lie on their other side, then lie on their back, and then go through a couple more cycles of lying on alternate sides before finally lying on their stomach. Thankfully, I still covered all the strength testing that I had planned. Or so I thought.

After the end of the patient evaluation portion of the exam, I had a little bit of time to document and finish a reflection form. On every other LPE, my mind was disorganized, and my trains of thought were haphazard threads being cobbled together. This time was different, and I could sense it. I had been reflecting on multiple levels during my documentation time and throughout the evaluation. With this, my trains of thought seemed to be more like threads woven together in a more organized, logical stream.

I met with Cathy and Dean in a conference room for the final oral defense. As we proceeded through the oral defense, Cathy would ask each question, and I would answer each one carefully and thoughtfully. Each of my decisions had logical rationale backed by appropriate research evidence to support, and each of my mistakes was self-reflected upon with ways to improve and concrete strategies for implementing those improvements. All of my alternate options during the evaluation were also discussed, and I shared different ways that I could have improved on information that I asked, and exam measures that I chose. While there was certainly room to improve with my self-critique, I felt like I had covered most of the important aspects.

Dean asked, "What did you think about the overall interaction between you and the patient?"

"Well, I could tell the patient was a little apprehensive about the entire interaction. Even though it was ultimately well received by the end, I think that the combination of my nerves and the patient's uncertainty expressed through both verbal statements and nonverbal body language with the exam, kind of fed into the overall patient-provider dynamic."

He nodded in approval. "That's a very important piece that you picked up during the evaluation. If you can continue to read both a patient's verbal and nonverbal signs and thoughtfully act upon those signs when necessary, this will take you far into your clinical practice after residency."

For the majority of the oral defense, after each of my answers, Cathy would ask Dean if he had any additional questions to add, and he did not for the most part as my answers seemed to be covering the content that he had questions about.

Dean did have one question for me though. With a twinkle in

THE FINAL LIVE PATIENT EXAMINATION

his eyes, he asked, "So Derek, did you check the strength of the patient's right gluteus medius?"

I froze. The gears in my mind began to spin. There's no way I forgot to check something that simple, right? So why was Dean asking? Did I forget to check? I checked it, right? Something's wrong if Dean is asking? My mind replayed the physical examination, taking notes on the strength testing portion when my patient spent about a minute or two rolling around on the table. I had planned to do strength testing for the quadriceps, the gluteus maximus and gluteus medius muscles on both the left and right side. I methodically started to check off each test in my head.

Right quadriceps? Check
Left quadriceps? Check
Right gluteus maximus? Check
Left gluteus maximus? Check
Left gluteus medius? Check
Right gluteus medius?
Right gluteus medius?
Right gluteus medius?

The realization started to dawn on me: I forgot to test the strength of the right gluteus medius so that I could compare it to the left side. Somehow my brain remembered a bunch of advanced clinical practice items but forgot to include a basic strength test that I learned how to do as a first-year physical therapy student. Dean stared at me, amused by the spectacle of me running through the mental gymnastics to come to the realization that I had forgotten to include this exam measure.

"Welll… I was intending to test their right gluteus medius strength once I had them lying on their left side on the table.

My original test order for efficiency was going to be the left gluteus medius, then the gluteus maximus on both sides, and then the right-side gluteus medius… Yeahhh… That was my plan…" Internally, I cringed. Whoops.

Dean shrugged. "It's not a big deal, you can always test it at your next visit. It wouldn't have necessarily had a major impact on your choice of treatment for Day 1. I could tell you were a little thrown off by the patient being confused about positioning themselves on the table."

At the end of the oral defense, both Cathy and Dean asked me if I had anything else to add. I had said everything I needed to say. Was it going to be enough? I sat in my chair, holding my breath.

Dean broke the news first emphatically: "You gotta relax, man! Overall, you did really well! You had a clear hypothesis list, tested it out with impairments, gave interventions to match, and rechecked it."

Cathy added to it, "I agree, overall, the LPE went really well, and yeah, you passed! Congratulations! Do you have any questions?"

I sat in shock for a second. Was this it? Did I really do it? It felt so surreal. I didn't know how to fully react to it just yet. After each LPE, it was standard procedure to submit the reflection form.
I asked if I still needed to submit a post-mentoring reflection form.

Dean just looked at me for a second. "No, man! This is your post-mentoring form!" as he waved his grading sheet. "You're

THE FINAL LIVE PATIENT EXAMINATION

good! Just submit something with, like, cats on it or something!"

We all laughed. As fun as it would have been to submit a form with cats on it, I still eventually chose to submit a proper reflection form as I felt like it was only right for me to finish out this LPE with no room for doubt. As for the scoring, the score threshold to pass this time was also 80%. My score was the highest score yet out of all of my LPEs throughout the entire year.

After the proctors left the conference room, I stayed for a moment. I felt a weight lift off my shoulders, and I felt light. All of my emotions came back to hit me in a wave. Tears began to stream down my face.

There were so many moments in the second and third trimesters and especially in the third trimester when I felt like I wasn't going to make it. That I was going to slowly burn out. That this wasn't the right career for me after all. There were so many patients who didn't get better. So many mistakes. So many setbacks. So many times that I didn't feel like I was still growing as a clinician, that I was making a meaningful impact on their lives. The tenet I set out for myself when residency began: to surmount a challenging journey of personal growth with the altruistic intent of working towards a best version of myself with a greater capacity to help with the healing of others through physical therapy… arrived just in time for my final Live Patient Examination.

As I wiped away my tears and stared at my reflection form, for the first time in months, I felt like I was going to make it to the end. I felt like everything was going to be okay.

CHAPTER 18

Goodbyes and Graduation

August 2021

After the third LPE, as I approached the last few weeks of residency, I started to say my goodbyes to patients. I knew that from a personal physical, emotional, and mental health standpoint, residency had taken a tremendous toll on me, and I needed to take care of myself.

As I said my goodbyes to patients and helped facilitate their transfer of care to the incoming residents, I started to note how much some of my patients not only enjoyed working with me but would truly miss me.

There was one patient who I had been working with for treatment of their elbow. I was in my final visit with them over telehealth and helping them transfer care.

> "So, unfortunately, I am leaving the clinic at the end of the month, so I'll have to transfer you to another physical therapist."

> "Nooo!! You're leaving!?!?!" The patient was shocked. "We love you, please don't go!!"

GOODBYES AND GRADUATION

It felt bittersweet to hear my patient say this, but I knew that I would not be able to stay.

"I know, we've done some great work together, but you'll be in good hands with your next therapist! It has been an absolute pleasure to work with you."

"Oh, but Derek, you've been soo helpful to me! I know you have to leave, but we will all miss you!"

We had a few more minutes in the visit, wrapped up the visit, and then the patient logged off. One of my colleagues who overheard the visit walked over to chat with me briefly. "You know, it seems like your patients really will miss you! It's been a lot of fun watching you guys as residents grow throughout the year." I suppose that from the outside looking in, it was more evident to the people around me to see that I was growing, and that sometimes it was difficult to perceive my own growth when looking inward.

Another one of my patients who I remember distinctly, came to me back in the Spring. When they first came to me, they were very depressed, discouraged by their hip pain limiting their ability to walk for more than a block. Over the course of a few months, we worked together for treatment of not only their hip, but also their shoulder and their back. At our second-to-last visit together, I shared with them that I was going to be leaving the clinic.

"You know, I've worked with a lot of different physical therapists at this clinic over the last few years, and you have been the best one for me by far. Do you know where you'll be going next?"

"Well, I'm not sure where I'll be next, I have to take some time to figure some things out."

"Well, whenever you figure out where you're going to be, I still want to see you for treatment. Whatever it takes, I want to keep working with you because of how much you've helped me."

I thanked this patient for their kind, thoughtful feedback. I knew that it would be some time before I found my next career step. I wondered where I would end up. I wondered if we would ever cross paths again. I also thought about how hard it could be for patients to find good providers who they genuinely connected well with. I hoped that this patient would be able to find the same feeling of empowerment in another provider that they found in their time working with me.

Later in the month, the residents were given a graduation ceremony for completion of the residency. We still had a few more days of working left, but all of the major examination requirements for us to complete residency had been met. The celebration was virtual due to precautions pertaining to the rise in COVID-19 Delta variant cases. Although I very much wanted to invite people to come for an in-person gathering, such was not feasible for the community restrictions in place. For the graduation ceremony, I invited my immediate family and my running coach. Also present at the ceremony were a few other faculty and staff, in addition to me, Mariano, and two acute care physical therapy residents. Each resident was introduced by a person of their choice. I chose Cathy to present on my behalf. When it was my turn to be introduced, Cathy first introduced herself as both the residency coordinator and the mentor for my last trimester before going into some words for my introduction.

"I actually still remember from last year in April, during the residency interview process, I was on the clinical interview panel and when we were asking Derek questions, he would do this:"

Cathy then sat back in her chair and put her hand under her chin in a chin resting fashion. I started to laugh, realizing that this was in fact a personal habit that had first developed through physical therapy school and carried into residency.

"We could tell that he was really thinking about it, that we could see him actively problem-solving from then on, that he was a thinker, and we were really impressed by it."

Cathy continued on with her introduction words:

"Throughout my time as a mentor for Derek, I could see the growth from him as he continued to be challenged, he would think and really reflect on the feedback that he was given. He worked very hard to apply this feedback, and it was very evident by the end that many of his patients truly loved him."

It was very touching to hear this. From behind my computer screen in my modest apartment where I was attending from, I tried so hard not to cry full-on. A few tears trickled down my face as I reflected on her words.

Over the year and especially the last trimester of residency, I had so many moments of feeling like the efforts that I was putting forth were inadequate, and it was hard at times to discern whether the rate of growth I was experiencing was on-track or not. Despite my struggles and setbacks however, I was able to grow immensely as a clinician and in the process profoundly impact the lives of countless patients.

> Cathy finished her introduction: "We've talked about how this last year has taken a big mental and physical toll on Derek. Hopefully Derek, you will be able to find time to rest, travel, eat good food, and recover physically and mentally as you prepare for the next step in your journey."

As Cathy stated, this year had taken a very heavy mental and physical toll on me, and I very much needed rest. After each resident was introduced, the faculty had each resident say a few words. I did not have anything formal prepared but took some time to say thank you to my family, the faculty, mentors, admin staff and friends who had supported me through residency and up until this point in my career. I honestly do not remember what I said, as my mind was still thinking about the year and third trimester in retrospect.

That evening after the graduation celebration, I typed another entry into my journal. I had some down time as residency responsibilities were now winding down, so I took some time to read through my journal. As I read through my entries, I started to appreciate that throughout the third trimester, there were many more expressions of heartfelt gratitude logged in the journal from patients than there were during the first and second trimesters of residency. In the day to day of being engulfed in the thoughts of my own perceived lack of self-worth in the third trimester, I did not realize how much I was still positively growing and genuinely making my patients feel valued. I knew for sure that this would always be a skill that I would be refining for the duration of my career, but it was evident in my journal entries that patients seemed to feel more consistently cared for in the third trimester and that I had grown in my ability to connect with patients. The week of graduation was perhaps the first week when I had taken time to look more in depth at my accomplishments.

My good friend texted me a congratulations that I felt captured the significance of the moment of reaching graduation:

> Yeah Tao!!!

> So proud of you man. You DID it!

> More importantly you learned to ENDURE!

I read the texts a few times over. The words succinctly captured one of the big themes of residency: cultivating the capacity to strive for and expand my absolute limits of professional development, facing a myriad of challenges along the way, and learning to not only gather courage to endure the challenges placed before me but to overcome them. It was about cultivating radiant resilience. Much had happened this year, but despite all of it, I was still able to make it to the end to complete the residency, and for that I was grateful. Graduation was not the end of patient care, however. After the week of graduation, there was still one last day of patient care to end the year.

CHAPTER 19

The Last Day

The last day of an arduous journey is inevitably sweet and bittersweet and sad. The last day presents a chapter closing, the sun setting, the shift of life from one stage to the next. A last day presents a chance to reflect on one's past time and memories. The last day of residency gave me time to contemplate my journey. In some ways, I felt even more uncertain about the world of physical therapy than I had at the beginning of residency. I had undoubtedly gained both knowledge and wisdom, yet the space of unknowns and questions about clinical practice had exponentially increased. Perhaps this would always be the case for the rest of my career: The unknowns and questions would always outpace the knowns and answers.

My last day of residency ended on a mentoring day, which I believe is the most fitting way to end residency. At the end of our final session, I gave a thank you gift to Cathy, a toy race car for her to add to her one-year-old's ever-growing toy car collection and thanked her for all of her hard work throughout the year supporting Mariano and myself through our year-long journey.

After we finished patient care, Mariano and I went to get dinner at some nearby food trucks. We reminisced about how far we had come in the last year and talked about the possibilities for the future. Mariano was going to be continuing to work at our clinic site, helping to teach the next generation of clinicians while continuing to explore clinical practice in his own way. As for me, I did not know where I was going to end up next. The future seemed uncertain yet bright, and the lack of a set plan felt very liberating as I felt that I could finally take the time I needed to take care of myself.

As the sun set and nighttime descended, we said our goodbyes and went our separate ways, both of us planning to meet up again in the near future to share about any exciting new career or life developments. It was the end of an era in our friendship and colleagueship.

Many of my commutes back home were filled with thoughts of tumultuous worries, ponderings about patients, and multi-level logistics planning to keep myself seemingly scraping by in my year-long residency. For the first time in many months, my mind during the commute back home was filled only with a sense of light tranquility and ease.

Epilogue

FALL 2021 –2022

On the very first day after residency ended, I slept for over 11 hours. My first meal of the day was lunch, and it took me almost an entire hour to make the decision on what I wanted to eat.

I knew by the end of residency that I very much needed rest, mental health self-care, and a chance to try to medically address my low back injury as it did not improve despite my best efforts to self-treat. I did not truly grasp the magnitude of exhaustion however until all of my fatigue crashed upon me right after residency ended. For the first 2 weeks after residency, I slept between 10 – 11 hours per day, and the most strenuous decision making I felt like I could manage was figuring out what I wanted to eat for lunch and dinner. It was not until I was about 2 weeks out of residency that I slowly began to feel somewhat normal again from a mental health standpoint.

Unfortunately, the loss of work-provided health insurance upon graduation further delayed my access to necessary medical care, negatively impacting both my physical health and my low back injury. An entire book could be written on the flaws of the current healthcare system in the United States, but I won't go too far into that. Suffice it to say that here I was a newly residency trained and credentialed healthcare professional with no way to see a primary care provider! Life ended up being uncertain and filled with more challenges in my post-residency era as I struggled with my long-

EPILOGUE

term low back injury before finally getting surgery to successfully treat the injury in the Summer of 2022. In the first 12 months out of residency, I only had the chance to work as a physical therapist for approximately 2 months. With the other 10 months or so spent outside of work however, I found myself reflecting more deeply on my residency experience, and through those reflections I began to find inspiration to share my residency journey as recounted here.

As Cathy had said to me during residency, there was still the hope that I would eventually be able to celebrate the hard work that I put into my residency case report. It was not until the Spring of 2022 that I finally had the chance to look back in depth on my case report and reflect on how much hard work had gone into its development. I decided to submit my case report for presentation at a national conference as a way to give it an opportunity to be properly celebrated as well as contribute in a small way to the physical therapy profession at large.

Fall 2022

Throughout residency, my mentors would tell me that as much growth as there is during the year of residency, the year after residency is even more interesting. The amount of information and feedback that a resident receives is far greater than the amount that they can fully process and reflect upon. One of the most important things that a clinician should leave residency with is the tools and ability to self-critique and self-reflect. In essence, the clinician should actually be able to mentor themselves by the time they finish residency. In the process, the former resident will come to appreciate how much growth truly happened as they get to explore clinical practice independently and without the stress of structured testing environments.

As I re-entered the world of clinical care fully healthy and refreshed in September of 2022, I began to further appreciate just how far I had come as a clinician. There were still plenty of uncertain situations and challenging cases to face, but I found myself much more comfortable and successful with making attempts to navigate uncertainties than the clinician embarking on his first few months of clinical practice within a residency. I also found myself granting myself more grace, working on acknowledging my shortcomings and spinning them as opportunities to keep improving. In the process, my appreciation for both the positive and challenging experiences within residency came to grow as well. I anticipated that this appreciation would only grow with time as I continued working with patients, and in the more distant future, supporting the growth of students and residents.

During this time period, I received news that my case report had been accepted for a poster presentation at a national conference. I felt a mix of excitement and joy at the news. During residency, I did not feel like I could give my work the proper degree of celebration, and now I had the chance to share a refined version of my work alongside a refined version of myself. Now that I was in a life space to re-dedicate myself, I stepped forward to take this opportunity to prepare for the conference.

2023

Throughout my first full year of returning to clinical practice post-residency, I continued to find moments to reflect on my clinical practice, the impact of COVID-19, and how different my journey as a healthcare provider would have been, had I not chosen to pursue residency. In short, many of the themes explored in the Fall of 2022 were appreciated on a much deeper level.

One of the major opportunities to reflect occurred during the wintertime at the national conference where I had been accepted to

EPILOGUE

present my case report. As I presented my poster, several students and clinicians came up to me, expressing a genuine interest in the topic, a rare spinal condition called adhesive arachnoiditis, and they asked me various questions. As I answered questions and shared what information I had, I thought about how this conference experience represented both a long-overdue celebration of my work in residency and signified a small, albeit meaningful, contribution to clinical practice. I found it rewarding to share my work within the larger community of future and current PTs attending the conference.

As for the COVID-19 pandemic, there was much that the healthcare world had learned since the start of the pandemic, and much more to learn about the long-term health and societal impacts of COVID-19. Every once in a while, a patient would share with me that they had previously contracted COVID-19 and that they were still experiencing various symptoms affecting their energy levels and their ability to breathe during exercise. I anticipate that I will have questions to ask and lessons to learn about the impact of long-term symptoms of COVID-19 on people in their daily lives. I hope that the lessons learned, and questions answered will expand my capacity to help people navigate life with long-term symptoms. These encounters still remind me from time-to-time of residency, a time when the world did not have effective countermeasures for treatment and risk reduction.

∼

Why do physical therapists choose to pursue a residency? Why do people choose to embark on difficult journeys? Why do people commit to challenges that expose and hammer their vulnerabilities?

My high school Honors English teacher stated that the purpose

EPILOGUE

of going on a journey is to learn more about yourself. Now that I am further into my clinical practice at an outpatient orthopedic setting with dedicated clinical education programs, I can say with certainty that I learned a tremendous amount about myself on this journey and that there is still so much more to learn and explore. I am by no means perfect with how I conduct my clinical care. I still make mistakes, struggle with hard conversations, and don't connect with every patient as I would hope to. Development and growth in the professional realm of clinical practice will likely occur for the remainder of my lifetime, a blessing that will keep life challenging but interesting.

I hope that my story is one that prospective and current PT residents find counsel in, a personal lens into the struggles and successes of pursuing a physical therapy residency. I also hope that my story is one that readers can connect with: one of gathering courage to face a challenge inspired by the *heart* of wanting to help others. The pursuit of residency, and the challenge of growing as a clinician in the midst of a global pandemic, provided a unique window into the lives of patients—people who sought comfort and guidance from me even as I navigated my own uncertainties about residency and the COVID-19 pandemic. Throughout residency and highlighted especially in the last trimester, the important theme of residency was that I was not just undergoing this year-long journey for my own purely self-centered goals, but also to invest in refining my clinical expertise to provide better care for my patients, to use this as an opportunity to put the needs of others before my own, and to do so in a way that would be fulfilling in the long-term. Perhaps what best captures my inspiration for pursuing physical therapy residency is a quote from Buddhist Master Shinjo Ito that I have reflected on time and again through the early stages of my career:

EPILOGUE

We cannot feel grounded if we live only for ourselves. Only when we also focus on the well-being of others will our lives be truly meaningful. Every day we can reflect on how we have been granted life so we can help to enhance the lives of others, rather than for the gratification of our own desires.[27]

When it really came down to it in residency, when my absolute limits were tested, when I was filled with self-doubt about the value of the clinical care I had to offer, what kept me grounded wasn't the goal of trying to just complete residency for myself, but rather it was the reminders from my patients about why I pursued physical therapy as a career, the reminders of why I chose to pursue residency. I was embarking on this journey to intentionally cultivate my capacity to bring a figurative *light* to future patients, and I knew that the care I had to offer them was precious but needed refinement. As I continue to progress further into clinical practice and life post-residency, I hope that I will keep building my own light to share with the people around me: colleagues, friends, family, and my patients.

ACKNOWLEDGMENTS

For every person who achieves a great accomplishment, there is an entire ecosystem of people who support that person and make the accomplishment possible. I can say with full confidence that I would not be the person or healthcare provider I am today without the help of my support system.

To start things off, a heartfelt thank you to my editor Jennifer Watson. As I navigated the process of writing and preparing my first book ever for publication, your thoughtful recommendations and expertise were invaluable to helping me bring out the best version of this book.

A big shoutout to my co-resident, Mariano Weschler is in order, of course. There's something special about being able to embark on a transformative journey and to do so with someone who mutually understands the inherent struggles associated with it. Mariano was a very solid, dependable co-resident and if I were sent back in time to re-do residency for whatever reason, I have no doubt that he would make a great co-resident once more.

Thank you to the residency director, Alison Scheid, for supporting Mariano and I throughout our journey as residents while challenging us to self-reflect on ourselves as clinicians and for allowing us the opportunity to undergo residency.

I cannot forget my mentors of course, as they were pivotal in my growth throughout the year as a resident. So, here are the Thank yous:

To Harvey Brockman, for inspiring me to become ever curious about the layers of complexity within the patient interview, for

ACKNOWLEDGMENTS

sharing your passion for plants: connecting the art of bonsai tree growing to the art of clinical practice, and for reminding me to enjoy the process.

To Kenny Leung, for our countless insightful conversations on career trajectory and moving the physical therapy profession forward, and for challenging me to critically self-examine the way I go about trying to connect with patients and making them feel genuinely cared for. That, and for the occasional random conversations about eating good food.

To Cathy Hoang, for your precise balance of challenging my clinical growth while also providing kind words of reassurance that I would in fact turn out alright in the end, even when I felt like multiple facets of residency and life were collapsing in on me in the third trimester. This is a difficult balance to deliver successfully, but it was done exceptionally well by Cathy.

Thank you to the various additional clinical faculty for providing their expertise throughout the year, serving as guest mentors, and for helping to teach the residency courses.

Thank you to the administrative staff for their hard work daily with managing referrals, scheduling patients, handling insurance, and performing all of the other tasks necessary to keep the clinic flowing. Good administrative staff goes a long way to keeping a clinic flowing. Thank you also to the clinic aides for the support with keeping things cleaned and for your work with patients.

Outside of the residency environment, there are plenty of people to thank for their support and words of encouragement. I can't list everyone's names here but there are a few that I want to highlight.

Thank you to my physical therapy school advisor, Betty Smoot. Our countless conversations throughout my time in school combined with your enthusiastic support for the various professional endeavors that I pursued during school were of priceless value to me.

ACKNOWLEDGMENTS

Thank you to my post-college running coach and good friend, David Marino. While you may have started off as just a fellow college teammate, you have become a pivotal support person in my life and have empowered me to grow as both a competitive runner and as a person through physical therapy school, residency and beyond.

A big thank you to my family, especially my parents. Thank you for supporting me constantly throughout my entire journey of going through school and residency as I pursued this dream and continue to pursue it.

Thank you to all of my friends, colleagues, and classmates who encouraged me to pursue residency, inspired me to challenge myself, and gave me words of encouragement throughout residency.

Finally, thank you to my patients for sharing your stories, challenging me to grow, and reminding me of why I continue to work little by little on becoming the best possible physical therapist I can be. Thank you for constantly reminding me of the importance of my work, and for enriching my life.

BIBLIOGRAPHY

Ito S. *The Light In Each Moment*. International Affairs Department of Shinnyo-en; 2010.

Physical therapy. *Merriam-Webster.com Dictionary*. Merriam-Webster, https://www.merriam-webster.com/dictionary/physical%20therapy.

Physical therapist. *Merriam-Webster.com Dictionary*. Merriam-Webster, https://www.merriam-webster.com/dictionary/physical%20therapist.

Residency. *Merriam-Webster.com Dictionary*. Merriam-Webster, https://www.merriam-webster.com/dictionary/residency.

APTA Physical Therapy Workforce Analysis. https://www.apta.org/contentassets/5997bfa5c8504df789fe4f1c01a717eb/apta-workforce-analysis-2020.pdf

ABPTS Certified-Specialists Statistics. *APTA Specialist Certification - Governed by ABPTS*. specialization.apta.org/about-abpts/abpts-certified-specialists-statistics.

Becoming a Physical Therapist. *APTA*. www.apta.org/your-career/careers-in-physical-therapy/becoming-a-pt

McKinley J, Rubin AJ. Coronavirus in N.Y.: Toll Soars to Nearly 3,000 as State Pleads for Aid. *New York Times*. April 3, 2020. Accessed May 17, 2024. https://www.nytimes.com/2020/04/03/nyregion/coronavirus-new-york-update.html.

Bowden E. Photo shows staff using trash bags as protective gear in hospital system. *The Hill*. March 25, 2020. Accessed May 17, 2024. https://thehill.com/policy/healthcare/489622-photo-shows-staff-using-trash-bags-as-protective-gear-in-hospital-system/

Federal Bureau of Investigation. *2020 FBI Hate Crimes Statistics*. The United States Department of Justice. Updated April 4, 2023. Accessed May 17, 2024. https://www.justice.gov/crs/highlights/2020-hate-crimes-statistics.

BIBLIOGRAPHY

Coronavirus in the U.S.: Latest Map and Case Count. *New York Times*. March 3, 2020. Updated March 23, 2023. Accessed May 17, 2024. https://www.nytimes.com/interactive/2021/us/covid-cases.html

U.S. Food and Drug Administration. *FDA Takes Key Action in Fight Against COVID-19 By Issuing Emergency Use Authorization for First COVID-19 Vaccine*. Press release. Published December 11, 2020. Accessed May 11, 2024. https://www.fda.gov/news-events/press-announcements/fda-takes-key-action-fight-against-covid-19-issuing-emergency-use-authorization-first-covid-19

U.S. Food and Drug Administration. *FDA Takes Additional Action in Fight Against COVID-19 By Issuing Emergency Use Authorization for Second COVID-19 Vaccine*. Press release. Published December 18, 2020. Accessed May 11, 2024. https://www.fda.gov/news-events/press-announcements/fda-takes-additional-action-fight-against-covid-19-issuing-emergency-use-authorization-second-covid

Wise L, Lucey C, Restuccia A. 'The Protesters Are in the Building.' Inside the Capitol Stormed by a Pro-Trump Mob. *The Wall Street Journal*. January 6, 2021. Accessed May 22, 2024. https://www.wsj.com/articles/the-protesters-are-in-the-building-inside-the-capitol-stormed-by-a-pro-trump-mob-11609984654.

Baker PE. Biden Inaugurated as the 46th President Amid a Cascade of Crises. *The New York Times*. January 20, 2021. Accessed May 22, 2024. https://www.nytimes.com/2021/01/20/us/politics/biden-president.html

Robbins R, Robles F, Arango T. Here's Why Distribution of the Vaccine Is Taking Longer Than Expected. December 31, 2020. Accessed May 22, 2024. https://www.nytimes.com/2020/12/31/health/vaccine-distribution-delays.html

Diaz, Jaclyn and Romo, Vanessa. "8 Women Shot to Death at Atlanta Massage Parlors; Man Arrested." *NPR*. March 16, 2021. Accessed May 22, 2024. https://www.npr.org/2021/03/16/978024380/8-women-shot-to-death-at-atlanta-massage-parlors-man-arrested.

Martin A. "New U.S. Covid-19 Cases Continue Overall Downward Trend." *The Wall Street Journal*. May 5, 2021. Accessed May 22, 2024. https://www.wsj.com/livecoverage/covid-2021-05-04

Mehta T, Mishra M. "Indian data suggests runaway COVID infections as deaths hit daily record." *Reuters*. May 19, 2021. Accessed May 22,

BIBLIOGRAPHY

2024. https://www.reuters.com/world/india/india-reports-267334-new-coronavirus-infections-2021-05-19/

"San Francisco Reopens and Expands Businesses and Activities as It Moves to State's Yellow Tier." *Office of the Mayor, San Francisco.* May 4, 2021. Retrieved May 5, 2024, from https://sfmayor.org/article/san-francisco-reopens-and-expands-businesses-and-activities-it-moves-states-yellow-tier.

Connectedness - Teachings by the Shinnyo Masters. *Oyasono.Online.* oyasono.online/welcome/1655

ENDNOTES

1 Physical therapy. *Merriam-Webster.com Dictionary*. Merriam-Webster, https://www.merriamwebster.com/dictionary/physical%20therapy.

2 Physical therapist. *Merriam-Webster.com Dictionary*. Merriam-Webster, https://www.merriamwebster.com/dictionary/physical%20therapist.

3 Residency. *Merriam-Webster.com Dictionary*. Merriam-Webster, https://www.merriamwebster.com/dictionary/residency.

4 APTA Physical Therapy Workforce Analysis.https://www.apta.org/contentassets/5997bfa5c8504df789fe4f1c01a717eb/apta-workforce-analysis-2020.pdf

5 ABPTS Certified-Specialists Statistics. *APTA Specialist Certification - Governed by ABPTS*.specialization.apta.org/about-abpts/abpts-certified-specialists-statistics.

6 Becoming a Physical Therapist. APTA. www.apta.org/your-career/careers-in-physical-therapy/becoming-a-pt.

7 McKinley J, Rubin AJ. Coronavirus in N.Y.: Toll Soars to Nearly 3,000 as State Pleads for Aid. *New York Times*. April 3, 2020. Accessed May 17, 2024.

8 McKinley J, Rubin AJ. Coronavirus in N.Y.: Toll Soars to Nearly 3,000 as State Pleads for Aid. *New York Times*. April 3, 2020. Accessed May 17, 2024.

9 Bowden E. Photo shows staff using trash bags as protective gear in hospital system. *The Hill*. March 25, 2020. Accessed May 17, 2024. https://thehill.com/policy/healthcare/489622-photo-shows-staff-using-trash-bags-asprotective-gear-in-hospital-system/

ENDNOTES

10 Coronavirus in the U.S.: Latest Map and Case Count. *New York Times*. March 3, 2020. Updated March 23, 2023. Accessed May 17, 2024. https://www.nytimes.com/interactive/2021/us/covid-cases.html

11 Federal Bureau of Investigation. *2020 FBI Hate Crimes Statistics*. The United States Department of Justice. Updated April 4, 2023. Accessed May 17, 2024. https://www.justice.gov/crs/highlights/2020-hate-crimes-statistics.

12 Coronavirus in the U.S.: Latest Map and Case Count. *New York Times*. March 3, 2020. Updated March 23, 2023. Accessed May 17, 2024. https://www.nytimes.com/interactive/2021/us/covid-cases.html

13 Coronavirus in the U.S.: Latest Map and Case Count. *New York Times*. March 3, 2020. Updated March 23, 2023. Accessed May 17, 2024. https://www.nytimes.com/interactive/2021/us/covid-cases.html

14 Coronavirus in the U.S.: Latest Map and Case Count. *New York Times*. March 3, 2020. Updated March 23, 2023. Accessed May 17, 2024. https://www.nytimes.com/interactive/2021/us/covid-cases.html

15 Coronavirus in the U.S.: Latest Map and Case Count. *New York Times*. March 3, 2020. Updated March 23, 2023. Accessed May 17, 2024. https://www.nytimes.com/interactive/2021/us/covid-cases.html

16 U.S. Food and Drug Administration. *FDA Takes Key Action in Fight Against COVID-19 By Issuing Emergency Use Authorization for First COVID-19 Vaccine*. Press release. Published December 11, 2020. Accessed May 11, 2024. https://www.fda.gov/news-events/press-announcements/fda-takes-key-action-fight-against-covid-19-issuingemergency-use-authorization-first-covid-19

17 U.S. Food and Drug Administration. *FDA Takes Additional Action in Fight Against COVID-19 By Issuing Emergency Use Authorization for Second COVID-19 Vaccine*. Press release. Published December 18, 2020. Accessed May 11, 2024. https://www.fda.gov/news-events/press-announcements/fda-takes-additional-action-fight-against-covid-19-issuing-emergency-use-authorization-second-covid

18 Wise L, Lucey C, Restuccia A. 'The Protesters Are in the Building.' Inside the Capitol Stormed by a Pro-Trump Mob. *The Wall Street Journal*. January 6, 2021. Accessed May 22, 2024. https://www.wsj.com/articles/theprotesters-are-in-the-building-inside-the-capitol-stormed-by-a-pro-trump-mob-11609984654

ENDNOTES

19 Baker PE. Biden Inaugurated as the 46th President Amid a Cascade of Crises. *The New York Times*. January 20, 2021. Accessed May 22, 2024. https://www.nytimes.com/2021/01/20/us/politics/biden-president.htmll

20 U.S. Food and Drug Administration. *FDA Takes Key Action in Fight Against COVID-19 By Issuing Emergency Use Authorization for First COVID-19 Vaccine. Press release.* Published December 11, 2020. Accessed May 11, 2024. https://www.fda.gov/news-events/press-announcements/fda-takes-key-action-fight-against-covid-19-issuingemergency-use-authorization-first-covid-19

21 U.S. Food and Drug Administration. *FDA Takes Additional Action in Fight Against COVID-19 By Issuing Emergency Use Authorization for Second COVID-19 Vaccine.* Press release. Published December 18, 2020. Accessed May 11, 2024. https://www.fda.gov/news-events/press-announcements/fda-takes-additional-action-fight-against-covid-19-issuing-emergency-use-authorization-second-covid

22 Robbins R, Robles F, Arango T. Here's Why Distribution of the Vaccine Is Taking Longer Than Expected. December 31, 2020. Accessed May 22, 2024. https://www.nytimes.com/2020/12/31/health/vaccine-distribution-delays.html

23 Diaz, Jaclyn and Romo, Vanessa. "8 Women Shot to Death at Atlanta Massage Parlors; Man Arrested." *NPR*. March 16, 2021. Accessed May 22, 2024. https://www.npr.org/2021/03/16/978024380/8-women-shot-to-deathat-atlanta-massage-parlors-man-arrested.

24 Martin A. "New U.S. Covid-19 Cases Continue Overall Downward Trend." *The Wall Street Journal*. May 5, 2021. Accessed May 22, 2024. https://www.wsj.com/livecoverage/covid-2021-05-04

25 Mehta T, Mishra M. "Indian data suggests runaway COVID infections as deaths hit daily record." *Reuters*. May 19, 2021. Accessed May 22, 2024. https://www.reuters.com/world/india/india-reports-267334-new-coronavirusinfections-2021-05-19/

26 "San Francisco Reopens and Expands Businesses and Activities as It Moves to State's Yellow Tier." *Office of the Mayor, San Francisco*. May 4, 2021. Retrieved May 5, 2024, from https://sfmayor.org/article/san-franciscoreopens-and-expands-businesses-and-activities-it-moves-states-yellow-tier

27 Connectedness - Teachings by the Shinnyo Masters. *Oyasono.Online*. oyasono.online/welcome/1655

Printed in the USA
CPSIA information can be obtained
at www.ICGtesting.com
LVHW091223091224
798490LV00008B/815